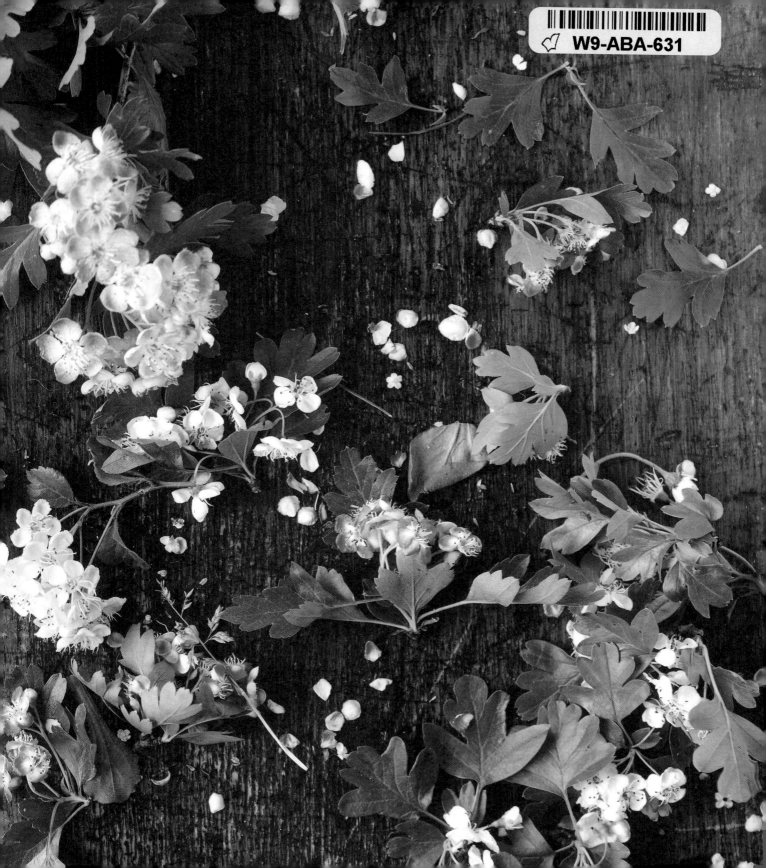

THE HANDMADE APOTHECARY

HEALING HERBAL REMEDIES

VICKY CHOWN
& KIM WALKER

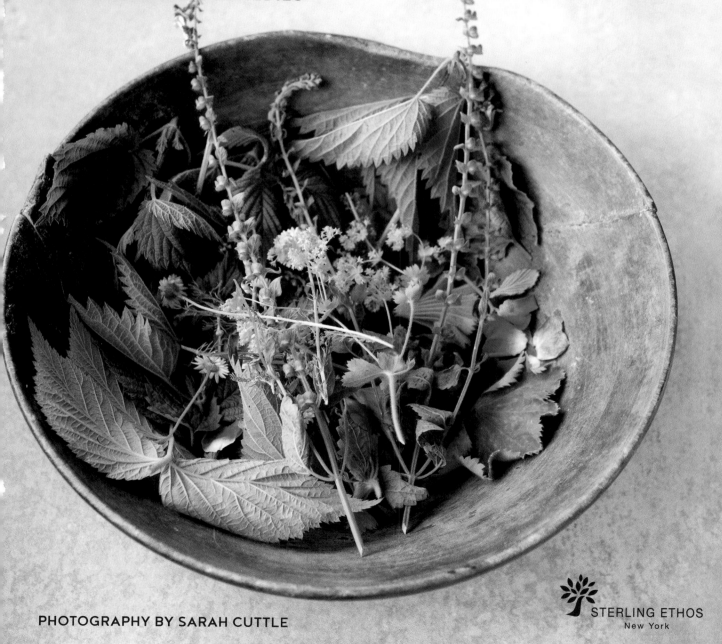

PHOTOGRAPHY BY SARAH CUTTLE

STERLING ETHOS
New York

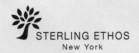

STERLING ETHOS

New York

An Imprint of Sterling Publishing Co., Inc.
1166 Avenue of the Americas
New York, NY 10036

First published in Great Britain in 2017 by Kyle Books

Interior text © 2017 Vicky Chown and Kim Walker
Photography © 2017 Sarah Cuttle

ISBN 978-1-4549-3066-2

Distributed in Canada by Sterling Publishing Co., Inc.
c/o Canadian Manda Group, 664 Annette Street, Toronto, Ontario M6S 2C8, Canada

For information about custom editions, special sales, and premium and corporate purchases, please contact Sterling Special Sales at 800-805-5489 or specialsales@sterlingpublishing.com.

Manufactured in China

1 2 3 4 5 6 7 8 9 10
sterlingpublishing.com

Additional photography credits:
p93: hoch2wo / Alamy Stock Photo;
p109: Bon Appetit / Alamy Stock Photo;
p121 top right: PhotoAlto / Alamy Stock Photo;
p140: Terrance Klassen / Alamy Stock Photo

To my wonderful parents Lyn and Gary, and to Cameron for all the adventures we have shared. Vicky

To my Grandmother Vera, who guided me, and to Ashley for his wonderful support and dinners, cooked while I typed late into the night. Kim

CONTENTS

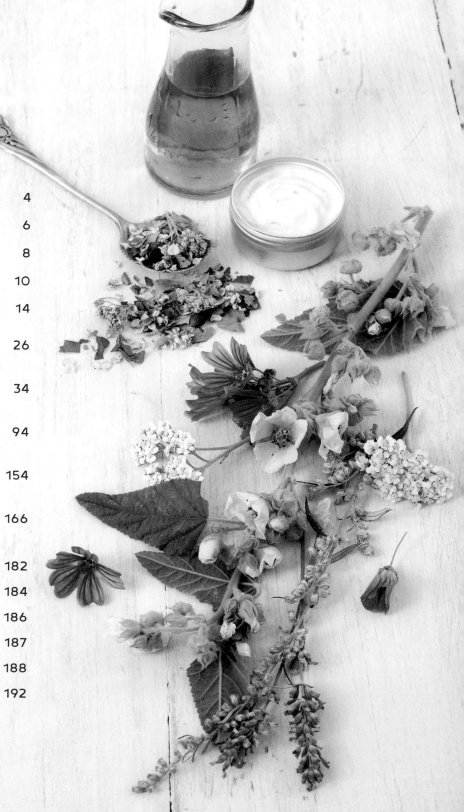

WHAT IS HERBAL MEDICINE?

Put simply, herbal medicine is the therapeutic use of plants and plant extracts to exert an effect on the body. Its roots delve back into time, with archaeological evidence dating to at least the Neanderthal period. Traces of yarrow and chamomile were found ingrained in the teeth of 50,000-year-old skeletons discovered in Spanish caves. These herbs have little caloric value, which suggests they may have been used for medicine. The plant-rich landscapes around ancient peoples not only provided food and materials but also offered accessible "pharmacies" to treat sickness and disease. Today, plants continue to provide nearly everything around us from food and clothing to medicine. Many common drugs are still derived or synthesized from plants; the contraceptive pill was first developed from a constituent in yams, and some cancer treatments come from yew trees (Taxus spp.) and Madagascan periwinkle (Catharanthus roseus). A constant stream of scientific research shows that herbal medicine remains a significant source of discovery to this day, with exciting developments in treatments for malaria, cancers, and antibiotic resistance. Using herbs at home can be as simple as a cup of chamomile tea for tummy ache or lavender essential oil to aid sleep. They can be used symptomatically, to treat and manage symptoms, and/or preventatively, to keep the body healthy and prevent disease. Herbs can be incorporated into daily life in the form of foods and teas and need not always be thought of as medicines but rather tonics to maintain a good state of health. When illness does strike, a well-stocked herbal medicine cabinet can provide relief for all manner of simple conditions and ailments. Herbal medicine is a holistic practice that considers many factors including diet, lifestyle, and medical history to get to the root cause of illness. For example, headaches can have numerous origins: digestive problems, neck tension, dehydration, imbalanced hormones, and circulatory problems . . . the list goes on. Reaching for a painkiller as a quick fix is sometimes necessary, especially when the problem is acute and you need to get on with your day. But true well-being requires more, taking time to be personally involved in your own healing process, making the necessary diet or lifestyle changes, and preparing your own remedies can result in more successful healing, particularly when it is long term or chronic. Herbal medicine merges the best of traditional herbal knowledge with modern scientific research and understanding of the body. Its great strength is its accessibility—it can be used by anyone with even the most basic equipment and resources; gathered from a nearby field, grown in the garden, or even picked up in the local supermarket. Herbs are quite literally everywhere, just waiting to be found.

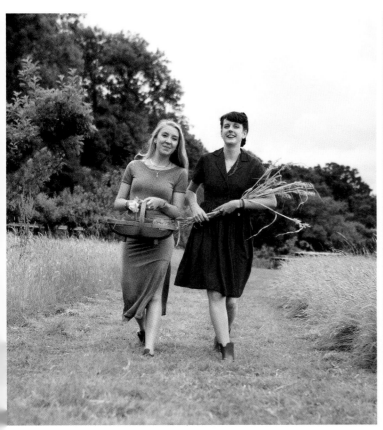
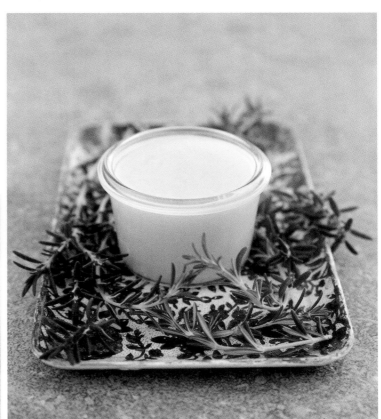
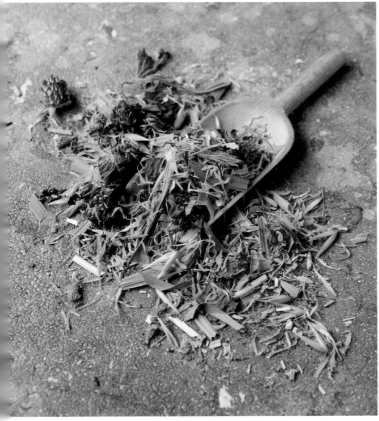
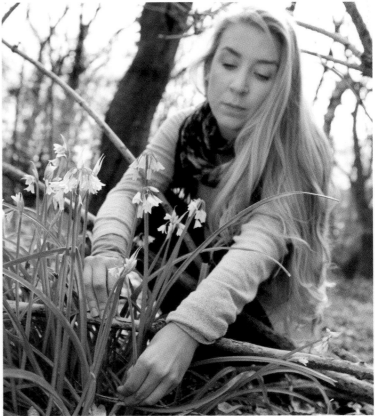

HOW TO USE THIS BOOK

This book aims to give the reader the tools to harvest and make their own herbal remedies for minor ailments and optimal health. It can be read cover to cover, used as a reference book for specific ailments, or used to find out more information about a particular herb alongside a good plant identification guide. We have chosen common, easily identified herbs that are often overlooked but have a long history of use as medicines and deserve to be embraced rather than weeded out. The way plants work can be complex, enigmatic, and hard to describe, so herbal medicine has its own language, referring to its effects as herbal "actions." For example, a carminative action helps to soothe the digestive system and reduce flatulence. Familiarize yourself with herbal actions in the Glossary on pages 184–185. Herbs are seasonal, so to benefit from them all year round, we have included instructions on how to prepare and preserve them. This book is full of tried and tested, practical recipes suitable for you to do this at home.

DOSAGES

While herbs tend to have fewer side effects than prescription medicine, they must still be used with caution. They are powerful in their own right and, like prescription drugs, herbs have specific dosages that must be adhered to. The standard dosages for herbal treatment in adults are as follows:

INFUSIONS AND DECOCTIONS 2 teaspoons of fresh herbs or 1 teaspoon of dried herbs to 1 cup (8 ounces) water, 1–3 times daily.

TINCTURES AND GLYCERITES ½ to 1 teaspoon in a little water, 1–3 times daily, unless otherwise stated (for any herbs that have specific dosages, this is outlined in the appropriate herb section). For treating children, see page 86–93.

FIRST AID

When emergencies strike, it is helpful to have ready-made remedies on hand. See the Herbal First Aid Kit on page 186 for ideas on what to keep in your herbal medicine chest.

USING HERBS SAFELY

When used appropriately, herbs can enhance our well-being, along with diet and lifestyle changes where necessary. Herbs can provide an effective and safe healing system for the whole family. Many can even be used long-term, where they can offer relief for prediagnosed conditions; however, for some conditions, particularly those that are chronic, it may be necessary to seek the help of a professional herbalist to get to the bottom of a longstanding problem. It is best not to self-diagnose illnesses. Instead contact a medical herbalist or doctor for assessment.

When taking prescription medications, seek advice from an herbalist before using herbs medicinally. There is a long list of herbs that are deemed unsafe for medicinal use during pregnancy. Some are listed below, but please contact a qualified medical herbalist before using any herb medicinally while trying to conceive, or during pregnancy or breastfeeding.

- Aloe (internal)
- Angelica
- Aswaganda
- Berberis
- Comfrey
- Elecampane
- Feverfew
- Ginseng
- Gotu kola
- Juniper
- Lady's Mantle
- Licorice
- Motherwort
- Mugwort
- Sage
- Schisandra
- St John's Wort
- Thyme
- Turmeric
- Wood Betony
- Yarrow

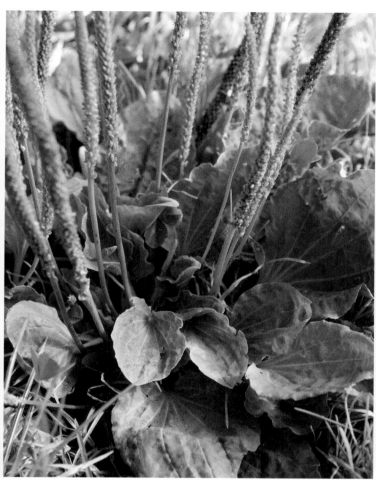

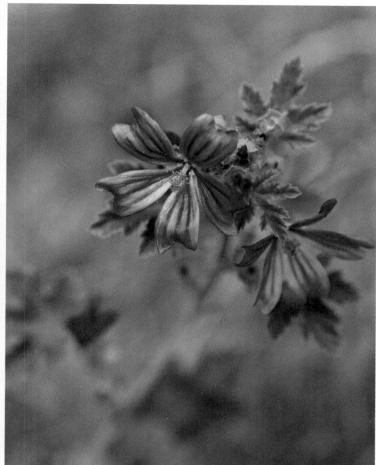

A number of culinary herbs should not be used in excessive or medicinal quantities during pregnancy either, although moderate amounts in food are considered safe.

DISCLAIMER

The information in this book is for educational purposes, to inform the reader about traditional remedies and approaches in Western herbal medicine. It is not a replacement for professional medical advice and treatment.

- *Do not use any remedies on children under the age of 2 years without first checking with an herbalist.*

- *Patch test any external remedies 24 hours before using to check for allergies.*

- *If you have any preexisting conditions, are trying to conceive, are pregnant or breastfeeding, are on any medications including but not limited to contraceptives, painkillers, and antidepressants, seek advice from a qualified medical practitioner and herbalist before you try home remedies.*

- *The authors and publishers do not accept any responsibility for loss, harm or damage from the use or misuse of this book or your failure to seek proper medical advice.*

Broadleaf plantain *Plantago major* (left) and
Common Mallow *Malva sylvestris* (right)

FORAGE

There are few things more satisfying than taking a long country walk, recognizing plants along the way, and gathering them for your own food and medicine. Get to know the plants in your local area with all of your senses—how do they look, what do they feel like, do they have a particular smell? Once you can do this, fields and hedges will no longer be a sea of green and plants will become as individually recognizable as old friends. Before you get started, however, carefully read this section, which lists some vital guidelines for foraging from the wild, safely and sustainably.

SAFETY

The number one rule of foraging is to NEVER consume a plant without double-checking its identification. Do not try to force fit an identification, no matter how much you may want a plant to be the one you are looking for. Always use a good guidebook and key out all the plant features. There are many poisonous plants in the wild that are easily avoided once you know them, so do not skimp on learning plant identification.

ALLERGIES Some people may be allergic to certain herbs, so be aware and carefully taste test a little of a new plant 48 hours before digging in.

GET A GOOD IDENTIFICATION GUIDE

It is essential to buy a good native plant guidebook and get to know your local flora before foraging it. Photographic guides are helpful, and learning how to use a floral key to identify the features of a plant is the sign of a competent and responsible forager. Most important of all, go on guided plant walks with a local naturalist, forager, or herbalist who can show you the edible and poisonous plants in real life, so you get a good feel for them and know what to avoid. Look for local herbalists or permaculture

groups for walks, or check out the Botanical Society of America (BSA). Also look out for local naturalist, foraging or botany groups.

PERMISSION

Please gain permission before harvesting from public or private places—foraging rules differ in every country. In many public open spaces, the flora is protected and foraging is prohibited for very good conservation reasons. Picking for sale in the UK is considered theft by the Theft Act 1968 (Section 4.3).

On private land, it's best to obtain the landowner's permission before foraging. Gaining permission also allows you to gather vital information, for instance, if any pesticides or chemicals have been used on the land. It is illegal to uproot plants on private land without the landowner's permission. Of course, it is immoral to pick any plants that are vulnerable or rare. Look after your green spaces.

IS THE PLANT CLEAN AND FREE OF CHEMICALS?

Make sure you harvest herbs that are clean, safe, and free from chemicals, such as pesticides and weed killers, animal or human urine, and anything else unpleasant that may have been left on them.

Don't harvest close to roadsides; the plants will be polluted by car fumes, fuel, oil, or rubber that washes off the road.

Take care when harvesting on or next to agricultural land or land previously used for chemical industry (for example, paint factories). Some old graveyards should be avoided, as potentially poisonous embalming fluids were used up until the 1800s.

SUSTAINABILITY

The issue of sustainability is particularly valid in cities: if even a handful of people around a single city park chose to go in and forage, there could be a negative impact on the park and its wildlife's diversity and health. Often, because of this, foraging is prohibited.

So what can you do and where can you forage? Try finding out if any friends have gardens or plots of land. Many areas also have local gardening groups or community gardens where you can learn to grow and harvest herbs. Additionally, it is in these community spaces that connections can be made with other people who may have good plant identification knowledge and similar interests to share herbal remedies and recipes.

When picking plants in the wild, never ever pick everything you see. Remember that plants, fruits, and seeds are important foods for wildlife. Leave lots for them, and for other foragers who may follow. Taking the root will kill a plant, so think carefully first.

Before foraging, research and educate yourself, respect nature, and remember you share the space with wildlife and others. Only take what you need, waste nothing, and help to promote the preservation and growth of more wild spaces for future foragers.

And finally, give something back: when you see seeds, take some and scatter them in other appropriate areas. Join a community group to litter-pick a park. Share your passion—inspire others to love their local plants too!

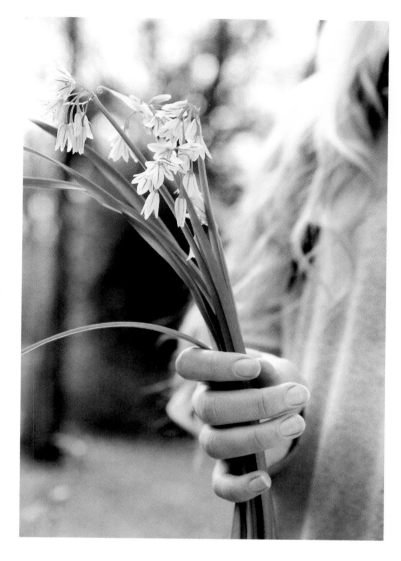

Three-corned leek *Allium triquetrum* (above)

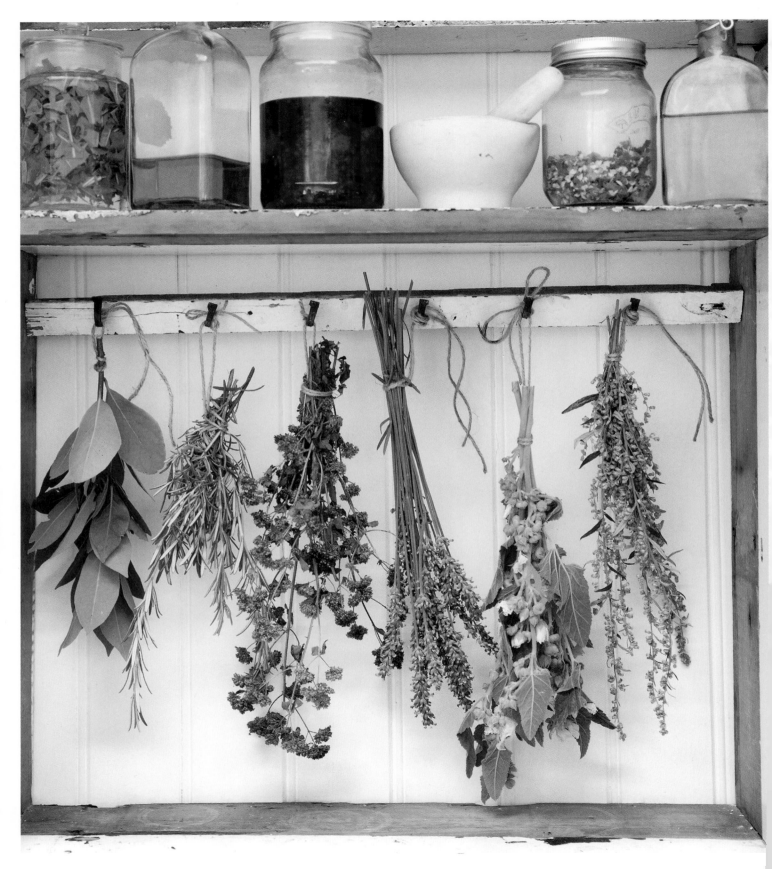

HARVEST AND STORE

Herbs are seasonal and should be harvested at their peak, to capture their healing properties when they are at their most potent. The simplest way to process and store them is through drying, ready for use year-round in infusions and other recipes. Here are some simple rules for when and how to harvest, dry, and store herbs.

GENERAL RULES

- Please pick respectfully, taking care not to damage or overharvest the plant.
- Always pick herbs on a dry, bright day.
- Remember to leave some for the wildlife and so that the plant can grow back for next season's foraging.
- Discard moldy, sick, dirty, or insect-damaged parts.
- Never pick a plant unless you are 100 percent sure of the identification—see page 8 for more information.
- Herbs should retain some of their original aroma after drying. Discard any that smell musty or off, or any that seem to have mold growth.

GATHERING EQUIPMENT

- Plant identification guidebook.
- Scissors or clippers for cutting, a trowel or fork for digging.
- Linen bags or a basket for collecting. Plastic bags can cause some plants to sweat and wilt, but are handy for picking things like elderflowers where you would like to keep the precious pollen enclosed.
- Gloves for nettle picking!

DRYING METHODS

However you dry your herbs, the drying area should be in a warm, dark place. Dry herbs out of direct sunlight.

STRING

Tie herbs in bunches and hang them up to dry.

PAPER BAGS

For plants that drop flowers and seeds when they dry, hang the bunch of herbs inside a paper bag to catch the loose parts and prevent them from dropping to the floor.

DRYING RACK

For smaller amounts of herbs, lay them out on a dish towel or newspaper to dry. Lay your herbs out with good spacing and no overlapping. For processing larger amounts of herbs, you can buy multilevel herb-drying racks made of netting. To make your own drying rack, cover a large wooden picture frame with linen, nailed or stapled on.

DEHYDRATOR

Electric dehydrators can be bought online for quick overnight drying, particularly if the weather is cold and damp. However, if you do not have a dehydrator, you can place herbs on a baking sheet in an oven on the lowest setting possible, ideally below 125°F. Keep the door open a crack to allow moisture to escape. This may take a few hours. Check the herbs regularly and turn if needed. Herbs will be ready when they are hardened but not burnt to a crisp. This method is particularly useful for thicker parts such as roots, stems, fruits, and seeds.

AERIAL PARTS—LEAVES AND FLOWERS

WHEN Many flowering herbs will be at their best between early spring and the end of summer.

Leaves should be harvested just before or as the herb comes into flower.

Flowers should be harvested within a couple of days of opening and before they wilt or go to seed.

As plants begin to die back, the medicinal properties will have reduced—the plant is now putting its energy back into the root or seed.

PROCESSING Dry herbs on a drying rack or in small bunches by tying stems together with string and hanging them upside down. They will be fully dry when they feel crunchy and can be crushed or crumbled between the fingers. Aromatic plants can be delicate, so avoid dehydrator or oven methods.

STORAGE After drying, store the herbs as they are in paper bags, or run your fingers up the stems toward the flower heads to strip the useful leaves and flowers. These can then be stored in airtight jars for a longer shelf life. Crushing or crumbling plants causes some chemicals to break down quicker, so store leaves and flowers as whole as possible. Aerial parts will keep for up to 1 year, but the more aromatic the herb, the less shelf life it may have. If it smells stale or musty, throw it away.

FRUITS AND SEEDS

WHEN Seeds and fruits usually ripen from the end of summer to autumn, but with unusual weather patterns, they can often be found much earlier or later, so get to know the plants in your local area.

PROCESSING Make sure fruit is ripe and neither bruised nor split. For larger fruits, slice them thinly to enable swift drying. For smaller fruits, lay them out in a single layer. It is best to assist drying in a dehydrator or very low oven. Most seeds are best when ripe and brown, but there are exceptions, such as nettle seed, which is best gathered when fresh and green. Dry seeds quickly on a drying rack in a warm, dark place, or in a dehydrator or very low oven.

STORAGE Most dried seeds are chemically stable and will keep for up to 2 years if stored in an airtight container in a cool, dark place.

BARKS

Never harvest bark from the main trunk of a tree as this can kill it. Bark can be sustainably collected for medicine from branches or saplings that are at least two years old—they're usually a pencil to finger thickness in size. This enables maximum return for effort, as smaller/younger branches are more difficult to handle. Fresh branches should be damp and greenish underneath the bark. Avoid if the branch is dry and easy to snap—this means the branch is dead.

WHEN Bark is usually gathered in the early spring as the sap rises, or in the autumn as the sap settles down and the tree gets ready to rest.

PROCESSING Prune tree branches in long lengths or gather saplings from the base of the tree, thinning out the "competition" and helping the main tree to grow.

Take the branches and then, with a knife or potato peeler, carefully strip sections of bark away from you as if peeling a vegetable. Cut these into equal-size pieces and dry evenly on a drying rack, or in a dehydrator or very low oven.

STORAGE Barks are stable in nature and will keep for up to 2 years if stored in an airtight container in a cool, dark place.

ROOTS

In the wild, "rooty" plants love to anchor themselves firmly in stony soil and are hard to dig up. Grow your own in deep pots of sandy soil and they will be much easier to harvest.

WHEN Roots are best harvested in the autumn, after they have had a summer of storing nutrients ready for the winter. Some plants, such as burdock, are biennial, which means they grow over two years and make seeds in the second year and then die. Harvest the roots of biennial plants after the first year when they are the plumpest and at their most medicinal. When harvesting roots in general, replant the "crown" of the plant just below the stem, or replant bits of loose, thick root, as some plants will grow back for the next year this way.

PROCESSING Wash and scrub any soil from roots. Peel, slice evenly, and dry on a drying rack in a warm, dark place, or in a dehydrator or at a very low heat in the oven.

STORAGE Roots can be stored for up to 2 years if stored in an airtight container in a cool, dark place.

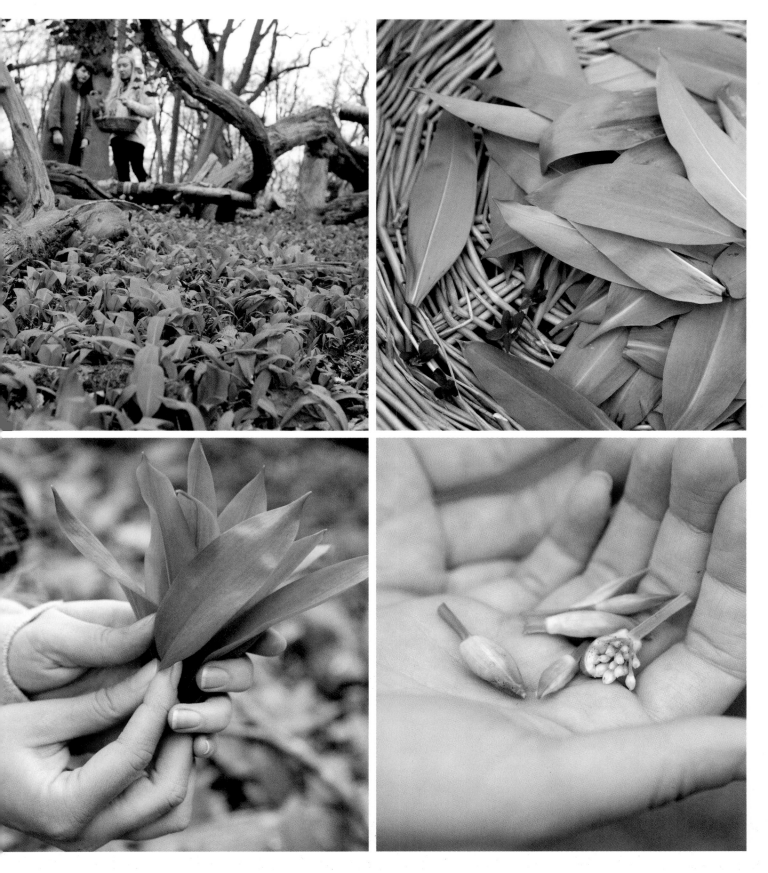

MAKE

Herbs can be taken in myriad ways—turning them into remedies makes them easy and convenient to use, preserves them for use throughout the year, and is also a lot of fun! The remedies you choose depend on what properties you want to extract from the herb and what condition you want to treat. For example, a steam inhalation to extract aromatic, antibacterial oils, a cream to soothe eczema, a syrup for coughs, and so on.

Always label and date herbal preparations, otherwise you will be left with a cupboard full of mystery remedies you will be unable to use.

STERILIZING GLASS JARS AND BOTTLES

Make sure all equipment is clean and sterilized before use. This is medicine making after all! It will help to extend the shelf life of all your hard work.

To sterilize glass jars and bottles, either:

Use a baby bottle sterilizing fluid, or

Preheat the oven to 250°F. Wash bottles and jars in hot soapy water, then rinse thoroughly. Place on a baking sheet or directly on the oven shelf and heat until completely dry, about 20–30 minutes. Make sure you do not put any plastic lids or seals in the oven. Simmer rubber Mason jar seals at 180°F to sterilize them.

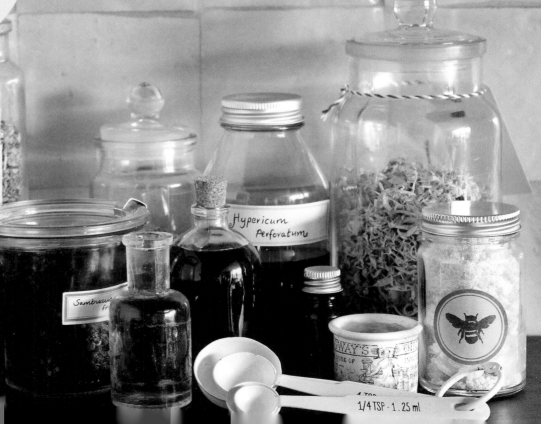

INTERNAL PREPARATIONS

INFUSIONS AND DECOCTIONS

Infusions and decoctions are an easy and simple way to take herbs. Infusions involve steeping herbs in cold or boiling water and are best for delicate herbs such as leaves and flowers. The plant chemicals in dried herbs are more condensed so use double, if using fresh. Decoctions are best suited to thicker, harder plant parts, such as roots, barks, fruits and seeds, which require a longer "cooking" time to extract the goodness. All infusions and decoctions can be stored in an airtight container in the fridge for up to 3 days.

HOT INFUSIONS (TEAS)

Use 1 teaspoon dried or 2 teaspoons fresh herb per 1 cup of boiling water and place in a teapot or lidded vessel to capture any volatile oils. Brew for 10–20 minutes, then strain and enjoy! Alternatively, use a tea infuser or cafetière.

COLD INFUSIONS

Some herbs extract well in cold water; for example, demulcent herbs including marshmallow root and mullein. Cover the herb with cold water in a bowl and leave to sit overnight. Strain and drink.

DECOCTIONS

Use 2 teaspoons of fresh or 1 teaspoon of dry herbs, crushed slightly, per 2 cups of water (some liquid will evaporate during simmering). Place the herbs and water in a saucepan, cover and bring to a simmer, then simmer gently for 10–20 minutes. Strain and drink.

TINCTURES AND GLYCERITES

Tinctures and glycerites are fluid extracts of herbs that use either alcohol or glycerin to extract plant chemicals into a convenient liquid form. Both are easy to make at home and also act to preserve herbs throughout the seasons.

TINCTURES

A tincture is a hydroalcoholic extract of a fresh or dried herb. Using alcohol allows the release of a wider range of plant chemicals than if using water alone. Making your own is much more cost-effective when compared to buying them ready-made.

Suitable alcohols include vodka, gin or brandy, which are strong enough to extract and preserve the herb. Medical and commercial alcohols, such as rubbing alcohol or methyl alcohols, are not suitable for internal use.

GLYCERITES

Glycerites use a similar extraction method as tinctures, but instead of alcohol, glycerin —a sweet tasting syrup made from vegetable oil—is used. These are ideal for use with children or people unable to take alcohol. Glycerin is readily available from pharmacies, but do make sure you get a food-grade one suitable for internal use.

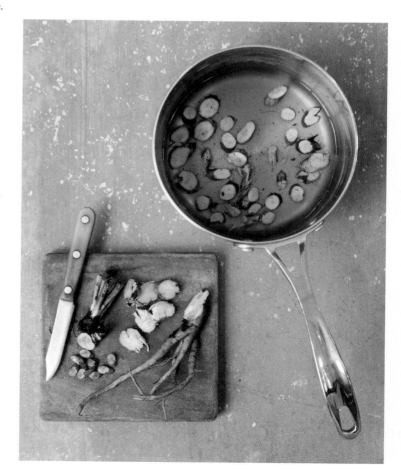

MAKING TINCTURES AND GLYCERITES

Fresh herbs contain more water than dried, so you don't need to add water, just the alcohol or glycerin. Dried herbs contain almost no water, and so can be reconstituted with just enough hot water to dampen them first, before adding the alcohol or glycerin.

Chop or crush your chosen fresh or dried herb and place in a sterilized, wide-mouthed glass jar to about two-thirds full.

Pour over your chosen spirit or glycerin until all plant material is fully submerged. If using glycerin, gently warm it first to make it runnier, and stir as you add it to the jar to release any air pockets.

Place the lid on, label, and date.

Store in a cool, dark place, shaking every few days for 2–4 weeks.

Once infused, strain through a strainer lined with cheesecloth or a thin dish towel, squeezing out any excess liquid.

Re-bottle in a sterilized bottle, seal, label, and date your finished tincture.

SHELF LIFE Keep in a cool, dark place for up to 2 years.

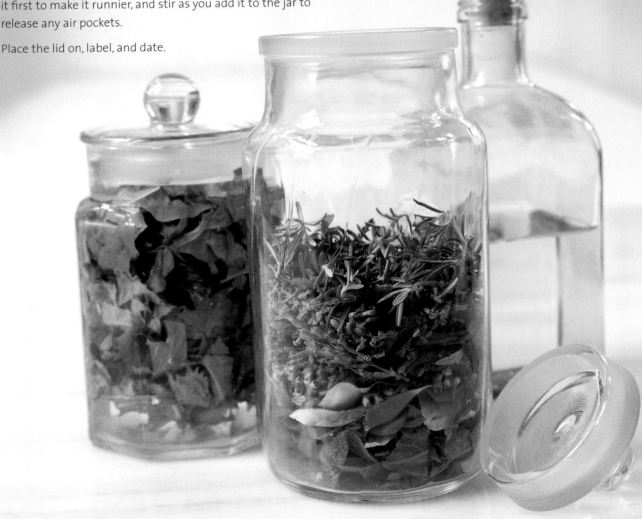

VINEGARS AND OXYMELS

The use of herbal-infused vinegars for healing is recorded as far back as 500 BC, when Hippocrates, the "father of modern medicine," recommended both vinegars and oxymels for persistent coughs and wound healing.

VINEGARS

Vinegars bring a cooling effect to a remedy and are useful in cases of hot inflamed tissues, such as sore throats or rashes. They can be taken diluted in water for internal use, or in baths and compresses externally.

Make an herbal infused vinegar in the same way as a tincture, but instead of alcohol, use vinegar. A good-quality organic apple cider vinegar is ideal and has been used for its health benefits for centuries. Infused vinegars don't have to be strictly medicinal; they can also be used in salad dressings, or dilute 1 tablespoon in a glass of fizzy water for a refreshing drink. Shelf life is up to 2 years.

CAUTION Neat vinegar can cause burns in some sensitive individuals; dilute with honey or water before use.

OXYMELS

Oxymels are a blend of vinegar and honey, which makes them more palatable. They combine the action of mucus shifting, toning vinegar with soothing and calming honey, ideal for respiratory disorders. Mix one part vinegar to one part honey as needed as a cough syrup or cordial.

GARGLES

Gargles are primarily used for mouth and throat problems. Use double-strength infusions and decoctions, or alternatively, dilute 2 teaspoons of herbal-infused vinegar or tincture in 2 tablespoons water. Swill or gargle for as long as you can, then spit out.

STEAM INHALATIONS

Steam inhalations are ideal for respiratory conditions including congestion and coughs. Use a few drops of essential oil or chop/crush fresh aromatic herbs and place in a bowl of boiling water. For adults, sit at a table with the

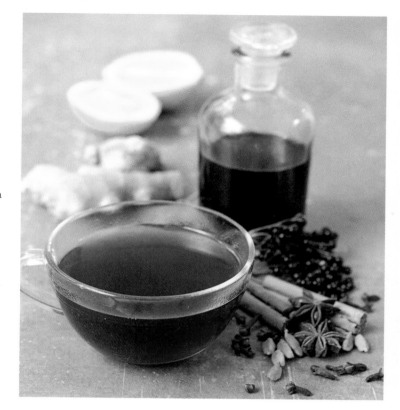

bowl placed in front of you. Place your head over the bowl (about 12 inches above) and cover with a towel to create a tent. Breathe deeply for 10 minutes, until the water cools. For young children, use a humidifier or mist vaporizer, or create a steamy atmosphere in a bathroom.

CAUTION If at any point you feel burning or discomfort, remove the towel.

SYRUPS

Syrups are another way to preserve herbs, this time using sugar, which makes them more palatable, particularly for children! Because they are thick, they coat the airways, delivering the healing properties of herbs direct to the area, making them ideal for sore throats and coughs.

Honey can be used to replace the sugar in syrups, but once it is heated at the high temperatures needed to make syrup, it will have lost many of its beneficial constituents and will have broken down into simple sugars anyway. The high price of honey makes this an expensive waste, so stick to organic unrefined sugars.

BASIC HERBAL SYRUP RECIPE

This recipe can be used for any type of herbal infusion or decoction and works well for making soothing cough remedies.

1³/₄ ounces dried or 3¹/₂ ounces fresh herb
unrefined light or dark brown sugar

First infuse or decoct your chosen herb in 2¹/₂ cups water, as described in the Infusion and Decoction section (see page 15).

Measure out the strained liquid, then for every 1 cup of juice, add 1 cup of sugar and place both in a pan. Heat gently, stirring until the sugar has dissolved, then bring to a simmer and simmer gently for 10–20 minutes, stirring gently until thickened. (You can use less sugar, up to half the amount, but it won't preserve for as long.)

Remove from the heat and leave to cool slightly, then pour into sterilized bottles, seal, label, and date.

TIP For extra preservation and to balance out the sweetness of a syrup, you can stir in 1–2 teaspoons of citric acid at the end of the recipe.

SHELF LIFE Keep in a cool, dark place for up to 1 year. Once opened, store in the fridge and use within 2 months.

SUGAR-FREE FRUIT SYRUP

A rob is a really thick syrup that can have a jelly-like consistency, depending on the pectin content of the fruits used. This recipe is not strictly sugar-free, because it is made with fruits and uses their own natural sugars as a preservative.

1 pound fresh fruit, such as elderberries, rosehips, raspberries, or blackberries
1 cinnamon stick
a few whole cloves
1 star anise
¹/₂-inch piece of fresh ginger

Strip all the berries or fruits from their stems, then wash and drain. Place in a saucepan with enough water to cover (about ¹/₂ cup—you need to add enough water to keep the fruits from sticking to the bottom of the pan and aid them in releasing their juices). Bring to a boil, then simmer, uncovered, for about 20 minutes, until the berries or fruit are soft, stirring occasionally.

Remove from the heat, then squash the berries or fruit with a potato masher to break them open. Strain the mixture through a cheesecloth-lined strainer set over a bowl (this is particularly important in the case of rosehips, as they contain fine hairs that could cause irritation when taken internally).

Pour the strained liquid back into the rinsed-out saucepan, along with all the spices. Simmer, uncovered, over very low heat until the liquid has reduced by half, about 30–45 minutes. Strain again, then pour the hot liquid into sterilized, wide-mouthed jars. Seal, label, and date. Once cool, store in the fridge.

To use, stir a teaspoonful into a hot drink, as and when needed.

SHELF LIFE Keep in the fridge for up to 6 months. Once opened, keep refrigerated and use within 2 weeks.

HONEYS

Honey extracts both the water- and oil-based constituents from herbs. You can make no-heat "syrups" by infusing herbs directly in honey. Because it isn't heated, it maintains honey's beneficial healing enzymes, pollen, antioxidants, and propolis. If you want to store herbal honeys for a long time, it is best to use dried herbs, as there may be a risk of bacterial contamination with fresh.

HERBAL HONEY

Place the herb in a sterilized jar and cover with raw honey.

Be patient and allow time for the air bubbles to come out by gently turning the jar (use a long thin spoon or chopstick to help). Seal the jar, label, and date, then leave in a cool, dark place for up to 1 month before use, turning the jar every day. Strain into another sterilized jar before use; seal, label, and date.

To use, take 1 teaspoon of honey a day. This can be taken straight from the spoon, added to drinks, or mixed into yogurt or oatmeal. For acute illness, such as a cough or sore throat, take 1–2 teaspoons as you would a cough syrup, up to 3 times a day.

SHELF LIFE Keep dried herbal honey in a cool, dark place for up to 1 year, and fresh herbal honey for up to 6 months.

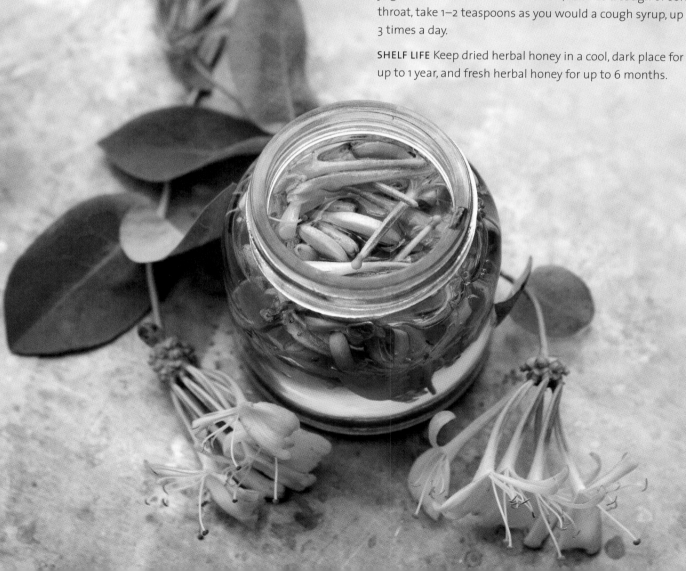

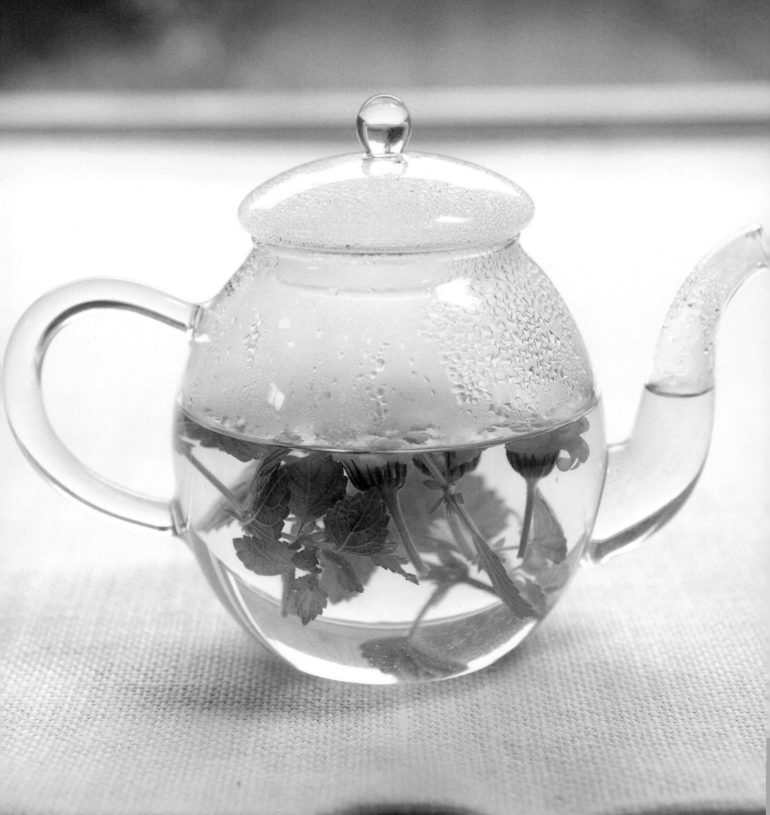

EXTERNAL PREPARATIONS

HERBAL BATHS

A wonderfully relaxing way to take herbs medicinally is in a bath. Some plant chemicals can be absorbed through the skin, and in the past, this was a popular way to administer herbs to patients.

Using herbal infusions in a bath is ideal for relaxation and many skin conditions. Shallow sitz baths are great for soothing urinary infections, menstrual issues, and injuries to tissues (such as after childbirth).

There are various ways to use herbs in the bath; you can sprinkle them in, but this is messy and can block the plumbing (tip: use a strainer to scoop out the floating pieces before draining). Many people advocate placing the herbs in a sock or a stocking, like a big teabag, and allowing them to bob around the bath. However, as the ideal bath temperature is around body temperature, this will not allow the extraction of the beneficial herbal magic. The answer? Make a big, extra strong pot of herbal infusion and add it to the bathwater before you get in (remember to check the temperature before you do so, though!). This final method allows you to get a strong dose and also saves the cleanup.

COMPRESSES AND POULTICES

Double-strength infusions can be used externally. Soak bandages to make a compress for strains, sprains, swellings, and wounds. Alternatively, you can soften the herbs with hot water, place between two bandages, and lay it on the area. This is known as a poultice. Whichever method you choose, leave the bandage on the affected area and cover with a warm blanket or towel, while resting with it in place for 30 minutes. Apply up to twice a day.

OILS AND BALMS

Infusing oils with herbal materials allows you to extract the medicinal qualities of herbs for external use. You should not take herbal oils made with fresh herbs internally due to the risk of botulism; placing water-containing herbs in an oily, oxygen-free environment can, in rare cases, cause the growth of this toxic bacteria.

Infused oils differ from essential oils, which are the volatile oil-based chemicals of aromatic plants that have usually been extracted by distillation, leaving a strong, concentrated aromatic oil. Essential oils need diluting before application to the skin because they can cause allergies or burns (10–20 drops in ½ cup base oil).

Herbal-infused oils can be used simply to massage on affected areas or as a base to create ointments, balms, and creams.

TYPES OF OILS FOR USE

Any pressed oil will suffice, but some impart their own healing qualities. Traditionally animal lard or butter was used—try it out if you feel brave!

SUNFLOWER OIL—cheap and fairly neutral in scent.
OLIVE OIL—cheap, nourishing and good for those with nut/seed allergies. However, it does have a slight scent.
ALMOND OIL—excellent for dry and sensitive skins, with a light scent. More expensive than the two oils listed above.
COCONUT OIL AND SHEA BUTTER—these make the perfect balm consistency at room temperature. Infuse using the heat method for an instant balm and store in wide-mouthed jars.

Adding 1 percent vitamin E as an antioxidant will help prevent your oil from turning rancid.

HOW TO INFUSE YOUR OIL

Infused oils will keep in a cool, dark place for up to 1 year. Discard if the oil smells rancid. There are two basic methods of infusing oils, as follows.

METHOD 1: TRADITIONAL SUN METHOD

This method allows the herb to steep in the sunlight over a period of time.

sterilized, wide-mouthed, clear glass jar
quantity of freshly dried herbs
oil (see page 21)
cheesecloth-lined strainer
sterilized jar or bottle, for storage
sunshine

Half-fill your wide-mouthed, sterilized jar with herbs and then cover with oil, shaking slightly to get rid of air bubbles and ensuring all plant material is covered (material sticking out of the oil may go moldy and ruin your oil). Seal with the lid.

Leave in a sunny place and turn every day for at least 2 weeks, until the essence of the plant has transferred to the oil.

Old herbs can be strained out at this point (through a cheesecloth-lined strainer) and replaced with a new batch of dried herbs to obtain a stronger oil, if you like. This is known as a double-infused oil.

Strain through a cheesecloth-lined strainer into a clean sterilized jar or bottle. Seal, label, and date.

SHELF LIFE Keep in a cool, dark place for up to 1 year.

METHOD 2: QUICK BAIN-MARIE INFUSED OIL

wide, glass heatproof bowl
deep pan
water for pan
quantity of freshly dried herbs
oil (see page 21)
cheesecloth-lined strainer
sterilized jar or bottle

Place the heatproof bowl over a pan of gently simmering water. Make sure the bowl is able to rest on the rim of the pan and doesn't touch the water underneath.

Put the herbs into the bowl and cover with oil. Simmer gently (keeping the top of the bowl uncovered), for 2–3 hours. Do not allow the pan to boil dry; keep topping it up with water.

After about 2 hours, the oil should take on the color of the herb. Remove the bowl from the pan, drying off the bottom to prevent water contamination. Strain the oil through a cheesecloth-lined strainer.

Repeat the process with a new batch of fresh dried herbs, if double-infusing.

Strain through a cheesecloth-lined strainer into a sterilized jar or bottle. Seal, label, and date.

TIP Alternatively, you can place the herbs and oil in a slow cooker on a low setting for a few hours, for an easy infused oil.

SHELF LIFE Keep in a cool, dark place for up to 1 year.

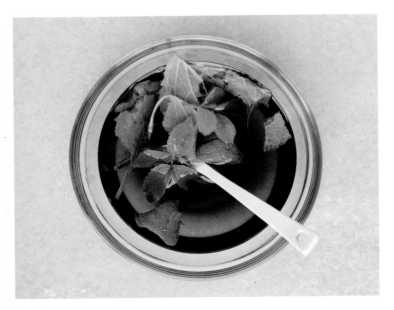

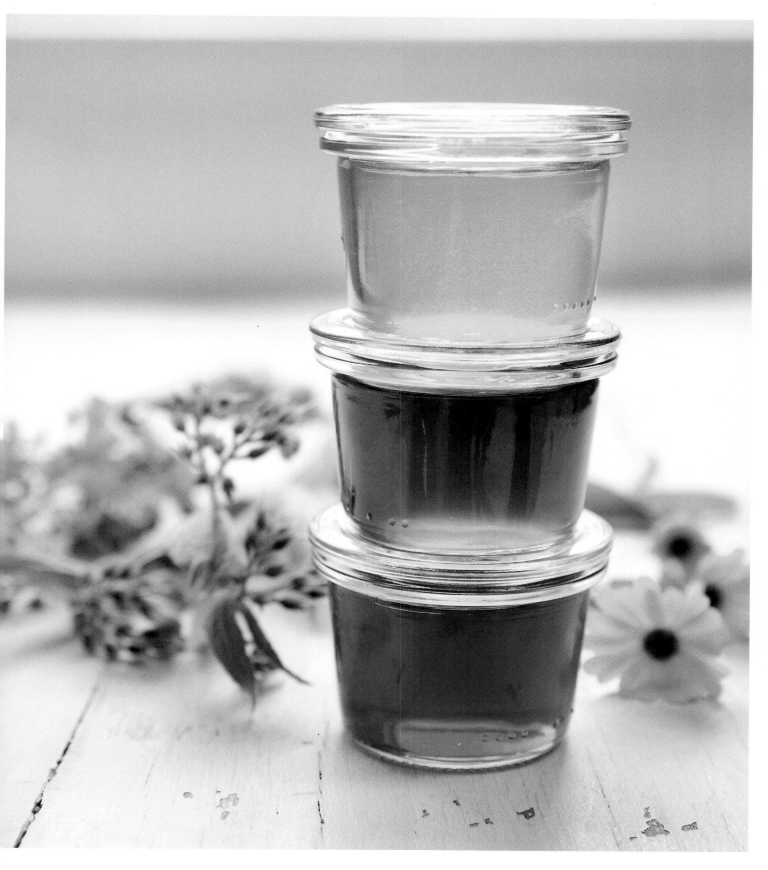

OINTMENTS

BASIC OINTMENT RECIPE

Ointments combine infused herbal oils and waxes
to create a firmer texture that is less messy and easier
to apply than infused oils alone.

¾ ounce beeswax
½ cup herbal-infused oil
25 drops of essential oil of your choice (optional)

Gently melt the beeswax and infused oil together over a
bain-marie, as described in the "How to Infuse Your Oil"
section on page 22.

Remove from the heat and leave to cool slightly, then stir in
the essential oil at this point (if using), before setting. Decant
the ointment into sterilized jars and leave to set in a cool
place, then seal, label, and date.

To use, apply as needed to the affected area. For external
use only.

SHELF LIFE Keep in a cool, dark place for up to 1 year.

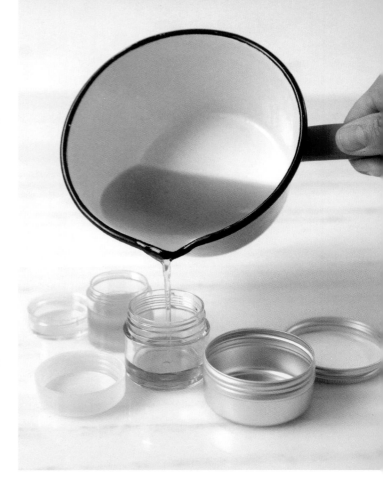

EASY VEGAN OINTMENT

Instead of using beeswax to solidify oils, you can infuse
an oil that sets naturally at room temperature (or in
the fridge in warmer climates), such as coconut oil,
cocoa butter, or shea butter. Infuse one of these oils
with herbs in a bain-marie, as if making an infused oil
(see "How to Infuse Your Oil" section on page 22). After
infusion, strain, then pour into a sterilized jar, seal,
label, and date. Use and store as above.

CREAMS AND LOTIONS

Creams and lotions are external remedies similar to
ointments and balms, but with a water component added.
This makes them a more cooling remedy for hot conditions,
such as itchy rashes, and can be more moisturising. They
are also less messy and absorb quicker.

Oil and water don't ordinarily mix, so to get your
two parts to combine, an emulsifier is needed. To make
a successful emulsion, the temperature of both the water
and oil components need to be the same; they can then be
blended together slowly – like making mayonnaise. Here
are two basic methods for making cream.

BASIC CREAM RECIPE

A useful base cream recipe to have on hand. Use herbal-infused oils, tinctures, infusions and essential oils of your choice.

⅓ ounce beeswax
⅓ ounce cocoa butter
¼ cup herbal-infused oil
4 teaspoons herbal tincture
2 tablespoons herbal infusion
1 teaspoon emulsifying wax
20 drops of essential oil of your choice

Heat the beeswax, cocoa butter, and oil together in a bain-marie, as described in the "How to Infuse Your Oil" section on page 22.

In a separate small saucepan, gently heat the tincture and infusion together, but do not allow them to boil. Add the emulsifying wax to the infusion/tincture pan and leave it to melt.

Remove both mixtures from the heat, then leave them to cool to almost room temperature. Use a finger to check that both mixtures are similar temperatures. The infusion mix may cool a little quicker; if so, return it briefly to the heat.

Gradually and very slowly, pour the infusion/tincture mix into the oil bowl, whisking quickly (a handheld electric mixer works best) until cool and thoroughly combined. This will create a creamy consistency. At this point, you can mix in your essential oil.

Spoon into sterilized jars, then seal, label, and date. For external use only.

SHELF LIFE Keep in the fridge for up to 6 months.

QUICK CHEAT'S CREAM (VEGAN)

This quick cream requires no heating and can be whipped together very quickly.

⅓ cup aloe vera gel
2 tablespoons herbal-infused oil
1 teaspoon herbal tincture
20 drops of essential oil of your choice

Place the aloe vera gel in a bowl, then gradually whisk in the herbal-infused oil, 1 teaspoon at a time.

Whisk in the tincture and essential oil until combined.

Spoon into sterilized jars, then seal, label, and date.

SHELF LIFE Keep in the fridge for up to 6 months.

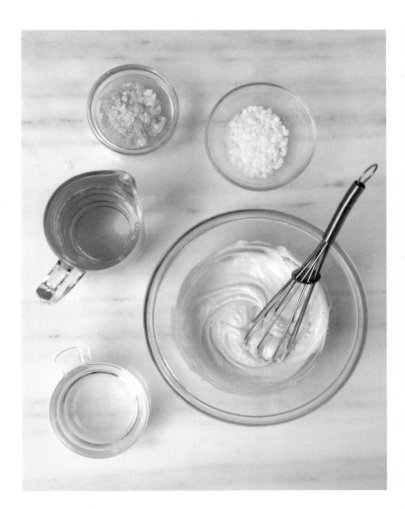

WILD GREEN EDIBLES

WHY EAT WILD WEEDS?

There is a fine line between food and medicine, especially when it comes to herbs.

The common weeds that grow in your garden can add a nutritional kick to your diet and come with a whole host of healing bonuses: they can boost your immune system, support the liver and digestive system, increase your energy levels, and much more.

Wild edibles are high in a range of nutrients, including vitamins and minerals along with phytochemicals. Phytochemicals (plant chemicals) are made by plants to protect themselves from bacteria, fungus, and predators.

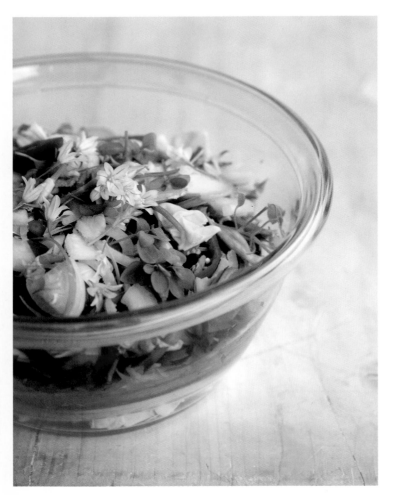

Wild plants are particularly high in phytochemicals, as they are more likely to come under attack from nature, unlike their farmed vegetable cousins brought up in protected growing conditions. Recent research has shown that some phytochemicals, including beta-carotene, lycopene, anthocyanins, and isoflavones, have potent antioxidant effects, while others are antimicrobial and can even prevent the mutation of cells.

A diet high in phytonutrients not only acts as a form of preventative medicine by supplying the body with a range of tools it needs to function optimally; it can also help restore health during illness. Take sulfur compounds, for instance; these are found in the Allium (onion and garlic) and Brassica (cabbage) genera and are antimicrobial, protective to the circulatory system and nourishing to the body as a whole.

Wild herbs are free, fresh, local, and nutritionally dense, making them the perfect medicine.

PROCESSING WILD FOODS

A good way to preserve the medicinal and nutritious benefits of wild greens is to freeze them for year-round use. You can do this by first whizzing them into recipes like herb butters, pestos and soups, then freezing in batches. Alternatively, juice them in a masticating juicer, or simply grind up your chosen herb in a blender or food-processor or using a mortar and pestle, then use a piece of cheesecloth to squeeze out the juice. Freeze juices in an ice cube tray for easy use, adding a cube to teas, freshly prepared fruit and vegetable juices (defrost the cube before adding it, if you prefer), soups or gravies.

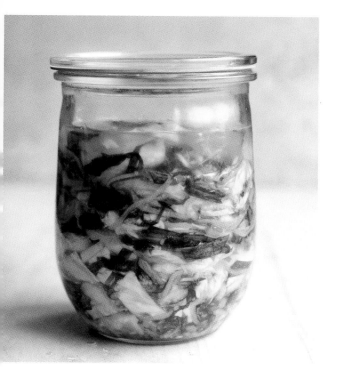

WILD GREENS KIMCHI

Kimchi is a Korean fermented vegetable dish loaded with spices. It is a great way to preserve nutrient-rich spring greens. The wild onions, garlic, ginger, and chiles are warming, antiviral, and anti-inflammatory; take a spoonful of kimchi to unblock sinuses and clear a stuffy head. As it is homemade, you can be sure it will be teaming with probiotic bacteria that can help to repopulate gut flora after illness or antibiotics. Plus it is delicious!

10 ounces mixed seasonal wild greens
2 large carrots
1 small onion
½ small head of cabbage
¼ cup sea salt
2-inch piece of fresh ginger, peeled
1–2 fresh red chiles (leave the seeds in if you like the heat)
2–4 large garlic cloves, peeled
a bunch of wild onions, wild leeks, or spring onions, finely chopped

Wash and thinly slice the wild greens, carrots, onion, and cabbage (reserving a few of the larger cabbage leaves for later). Place all the chopped greens and vegetables in a nonmetallic bowl, sprinkle over the salt, and mix well with a wooden spoon. Leave for 1 hour, then pour over 1 quart water. Cover with a plate that fits snugly inside the bowl and then weigh it down to fully submerge the mixture. Leave this to sit at room temperature for 12 hours.

After this period, place the ginger, chiles, and garlic in a food processor and blend together to make a smooth paste (alternatively, use a mortar and pestle and grind the ingredients together to make the paste).

Strain off the liquid from the wild greens and cabbage mixture, reserving the vegetables and liquid separately. Stir the spice paste into the vegetables, mixing well.

Spoon the mixture into sterilized jars and push down to release any air pockets. Top up with enough of the reserved brine water to submerge the cabbage mixture and cover each jarful with one of the reserved cabbage leaves to fully submerge the mixture, then loosely replace the lids.

Leave at room temperature for 3–5 days, then refrigerate (either keep the lids loosely fitted or be sure to open the jars every few days, as the fermentation can cause gas to build up, causing them to pop). After this time, the kimchi is ready to serve, or it can be left for longer, as the flavors deepen and the fermentation process increases with age.

To serve, eat on its own, or serve as a side dish, spread onto crackers, or stir into soups.

TIPS

For the wild greens, choose from a mixture of any fresh wild garlics/onions or wild spring greens (including ramsons, three-cornered leeks, crow garlic, garlic mustard, nettles, and chickweed)—see pages 28–31.

For an extra touch, add fresh hawthorn buds and young leaves, young linden buds and leaves, calendula petals (not technically green, but very pretty) or plantain.

SHELF LIFE Keep for up to 2 months in a cool, dark place and once opened, refrigerate and consume within 1 month.

Wild Garlics—*Allium* spp.
Amaryllidaceae

EDIBLE PARTS Leaves, flowers, bulbs.

DEFINING FEATURE Smell of garlic!

The *Allium* genus (garlic and onion) contains sulfur compounds, which act as alteratives, cleansing the blood and helping to clear infections, particularly of the respiratory and circulatory systems. These compounds also act as prebiotics, which encourage gut-friendly bacteria.

Wild garlics are much gentler than farmed garlic and are usually well tolerated by children. They can be used externally as an antiseptic for wounds; simply crush the leaves and rub over a cut for a first aid remedy on the go.

Use the leaves of wild garlic and three-cornered leek (opposite) like leafy greens. Add them to quiche, risotto, omelets, salads, pesto, and sauces to impart a mild garlic/onion flavor.

Wild garlic butter (see box below) makes a super quick and easy garlic bread or marinade; simply use it from the fridge (or defrost if frozen) and spread over a toasted slice of crusty bread, or use it to top cooked vegetables, fish, or meat.

WILD GARLIC BUTTER

For a delicious, luminous green Wild Garlic Butter, place a few handfuls of the washed leaves of any wild garlic species in a food processor, along with 1 cup (2 sticks) room-temperature butter. Whizz together until combined. Scrape the garlic butter onto a piece of wax paper, then use this to shape and roll the butter into a log, wrapping it in the paper as you go. Chill in the fridge until firm, then slice into portions. This garlic butter will keep in the fridge for up to 1 week, and can also be frozen for up to 3 months (defrost before use).

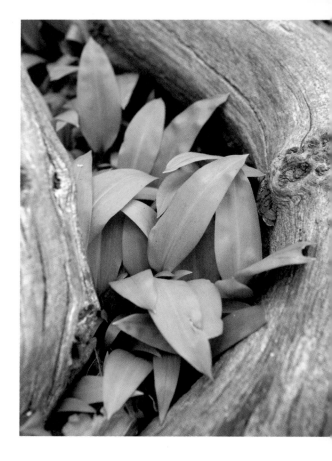

Allium ursinum

COMMON NAMES Ramsons, Wild Garlic

DESCRIPTION Ramsons are usually found growing in vast swathes in woodlands, carpeting the forest floor with their deep green, glossy leaves. The leaves are flat and paper thin and grow directly from the ground. The flowers have six sharp, white petals that grow in a roundish cluster.

CAUTION Ramsons have been mistaken for Lily of the Valley (*Convallaria majalis*) and Cuckoo-pint or Lords-and-ladies (*Arum maculatum*), both of which are toxic. Remember, ramson leaves smell garlicky!

EDIBLE USES Use wild garlic raw in salads or whizzed into pestos, risottos, or soups. The beautiful, star-shaped flowers have an even milder garlic flavor and make a beautiful garnish for any dish.

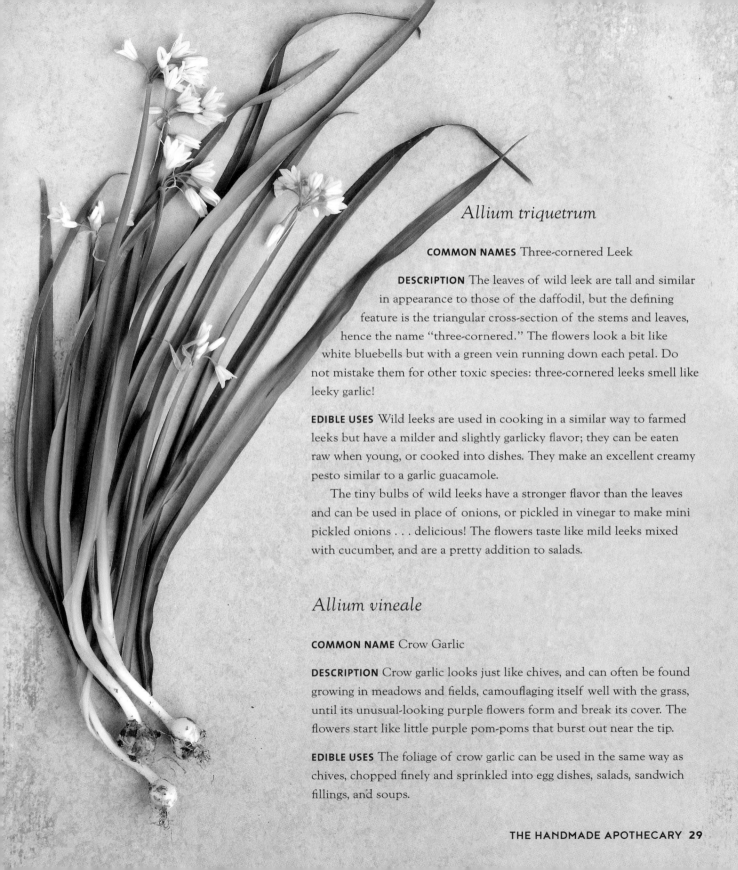

Allium triquetrum

COMMON NAMES Three-cornered Leek

DESCRIPTION The leaves of wild leek are tall and similar in appearance to those of the daffodil, but the defining feature is the triangular cross-section of the stems and leaves, hence the name "three-cornered." The flowers look a bit like white bluebells but with a green vein running down each petal. Do not mistake them for other toxic species: three-cornered leeks smell like leeky garlic!

EDIBLE USES Wild leeks are used in cooking in a similar way to farmed leeks but have a milder and slightly garlicky flavor; they can be eaten raw when young, or cooked into dishes. They make an excellent creamy pesto similar to a garlic guacamole.

The tiny bulbs of wild leeks have a stronger flavor than the leaves and can be used in place of onions, or pickled in vinegar to make mini pickled onions . . . delicious! The flowers taste like mild leeks mixed with cucumber, and are a pretty addition to salads.

Allium vineale

COMMON NAME Crow Garlic

DESCRIPTION Crow garlic looks just like chives, and can often be found growing in meadows and fields, camouflaging itself well with the grass, until its unusual-looking purple flowers form and break its cover. The flowers start like little purple pom-poms that burst out near the tip.

EDIBLE USES The foliage of crow garlic can be used in the same way as chives, chopped finely and sprinkled into egg dishes, salads, sandwich fillings, and soups.

Alliaria petiolata
Brassicaceae

COMMON NAMES Garlic Mustard, Jack-by-the-Hedge

EDIBLE PARTS Leaves, flowers, seeds.

DESCRIPTION A tall biennial plant with pointed, heart-shaped, yellowish green leaves. The white flowers have four petals, and the seeds are small, black, and contained in a long pod-like case. This plant is aptly named: the leaves taste like a mixture of garlic and mustard with a bitter edge.

EDIBLE USES It is a member of the mustard family, but like the wild edible garlics and onions, garlic mustard contains sulfur compounds, making it antimicrobial. It also has a bitter element to it, which stimulates and strengthens digestive function.

Add the leaves to starters and appetizers to prepare the digestion before a big meal. Use it sparingly when eating raw, as the bitterness can overpower dishes. Cooking reduces its bitterness. The seeds can also be sprinkled onto foods to add a fiery mustard flavor.

Galium aparine
Rubiaceae

COMMON NAME Cleavers

EDIBLE PARTS Top third of stems, leaves.

DESCRIPTION See page 114 in the Herb Profiles chapter for more details on this.

EDIBLE USES The whole cleavers plant is highly nutritious and has a wonderful lymphatic action, helping to clear infections from the body and improve a number of skin conditions.

Many foraging books and blogs recommend eating cleavers like spinach. While it has a beautifully fresh, crisp taste (a bit like cucumber mixed with new potatoes!), the texture is harsh; it is covered in tiny hairs that make it hard to swallow, even when finely chopped or boiled, so use it sparingly in food.

Alternatively, try the Cleansing Cleavers Cold Infusion on page 115, or use cleavers as you would wheatgrass in a juice; either as a shot or added to a fruit or vegetable juice.

See page 114 in Herb Profiles for more information about the medicinal properties of cleavers.

Plantago lanceolata, P. major, P. media
Plantaginaceae

COMMON NAMES Plantain, Ribwort, Broadleaf, Hoary

EDIBLE PARTS Leaves.

DESCRIPTION See page 130 in Herb Profiles for more details.

EDIBLE USES The hardy-looking leaves of plantain are edible! They can be tough, so choose the young, light green, fresh-looking leaves and use them in a similar way to kale. They are high in minerals, which you can tell from their rich taste and metallic tang.

See page 130 in the Herb Profiles chapter for more information about the medicinal properties of plantain.

PLANTAIN CHIPS

Make Plantain Chips by tossing the leaves in a little olive or sunflower oil, sea salt, paprika, and garlic powder. Lay them in a single layer on a nonstick baking sheet and bake in a preheated low oven (around 225°F) for 10–20 minutes, checking regularly to make sure they don't burn. They are ready when they are crisp. Serve immediately. These are best eaten freshly made.

Stellaria media
Caryophyllaceae

COMMON NAME Chickweed

EDIBLE PARTS Aerial parts.

DESCRIPTION See page 143 in Herb Profiles for more details.

EDIBLE USES Chickweed is the perfect salad herb; it is mild, juicy, fresh, and slightly salty. The only problem is finding a patch that is far from pollution and dog pee! If you have the space, leave a clump in your garden and care for it with regular watering. It is a bountiful plant that can be harvested as a "cut-and-come-again" salad.

Use it raw or cooked in the same way as baby spinach. It's high in protein, vitamins, and minerals, including vitamins A, C, and B-complex, calcium, and iron. Its mucilage content also soothes the digestive tract.

See page 143 in Herb Profiles for more information about the medicinal properties of chickweed.

Taraxacum officinale
Asteraceae

COMMON NAME Dandelion

EDIBLE PARTS Young leaves, petals.

DESCRIPTION See page 147 in Herb Profiles for more details.

EDIBLE USES The leaves of dandelion are edible, nutrient-rich, and tasty; the best way to eat them is simply in salads. Pick only the young, fresh, light green leaves, as their bitterness intensifies with age. This bitter element stimulates the digestive juices and improves overall digestion. They are a good source of minerals and vitamins, including iron, magnesium, potassium, calcium, and vitamins A, C, and B-complex.

The beautiful yellow petals of dandelion can be sprinkled over foods, added to scones and cakes, or made into an edible flower salad. Simply pluck the petals from the base of the flower and use fresh, otherwise they turn into fluff.

See page 147 in Herb Profiles for more information about the medicinal properties of dandelion.

Urtica dioica
Urticaceae

COMMON NAMES Nettle, Stinging Nettle

EDIBLE PARTS Young leaves, seeds.

DESCRIPTION See page 150 in Herb Profiles for more details.

EDIBLE USES Nettles are a nutritional powerhouse, high in minerals, vitamins C and E, antioxidant carotenoids, and protein. Only harvest the youngest, freshest, top 2–3 sets of leaves, as these are the most tender. Do not harvest the leaves after nettles have flowered.

Nettles are best finely chopped or blended into soups and pesto, as they have a rough texture. Some guidebooks even advise eating nettle leaves raw, but we wouldn't recommend this—it hurts! Don't worry, stings are broken down with cooking and blending.

The seeds are considered a superfood, packed with essential fatty acids, protein, minerals, and vitamins. They are also powerful adaptogens, supporting the adrenal glands and body in times of increased stress. Add them to smoothies, soups, and baking, or try the Energy Balls on page 66. Use the seeds fresh or freshly frozen, as they do not store well.

See page 150 in Herb Profiles for more information about the medicinal properties of nettles.

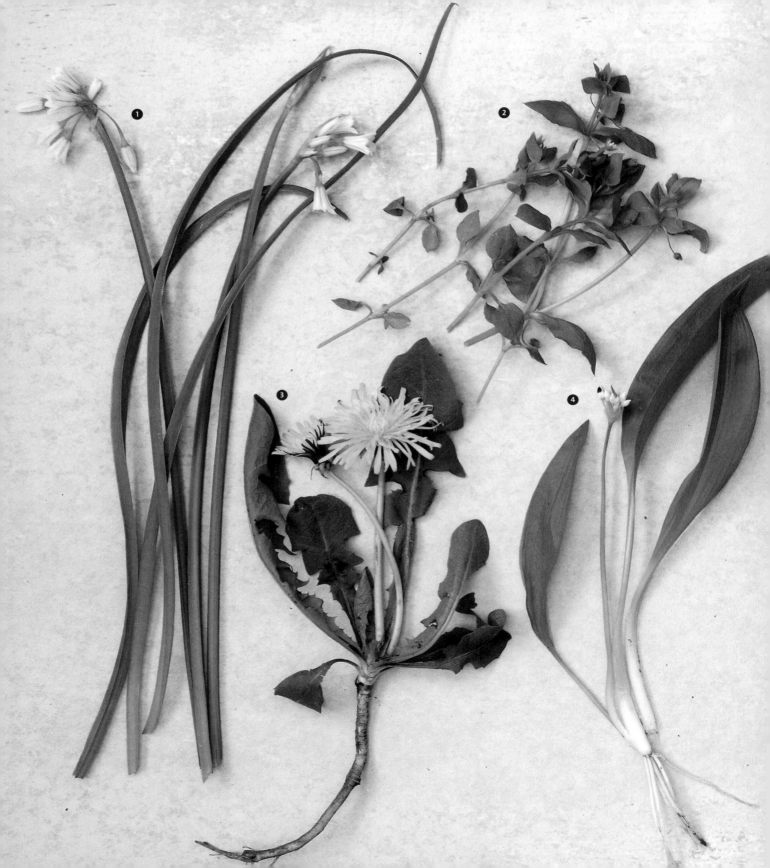

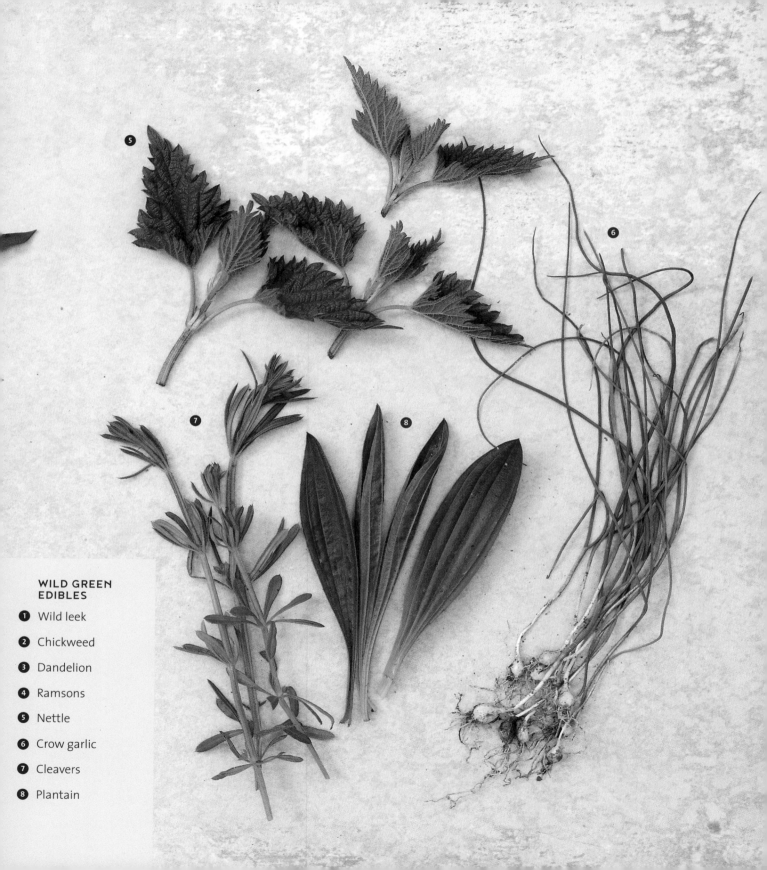

WILD GREEN EDIBLES

1. Wild leek
2. Chickweed
3. Dandelion
4. Ramsons
5. Nettle
6. Crow garlic
7. Cleavers
8. Plantain

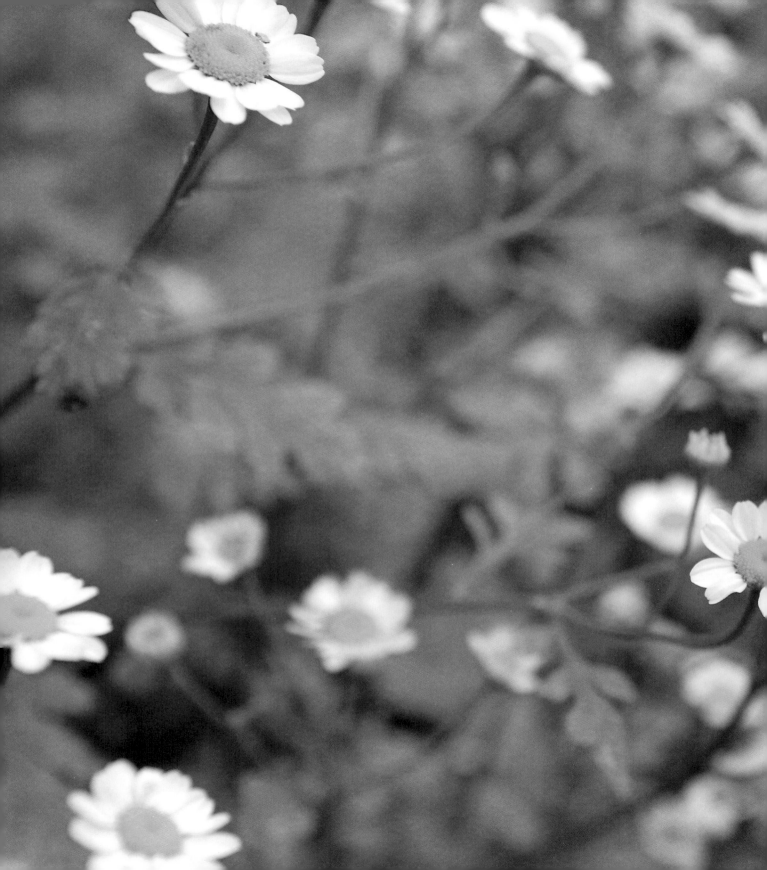

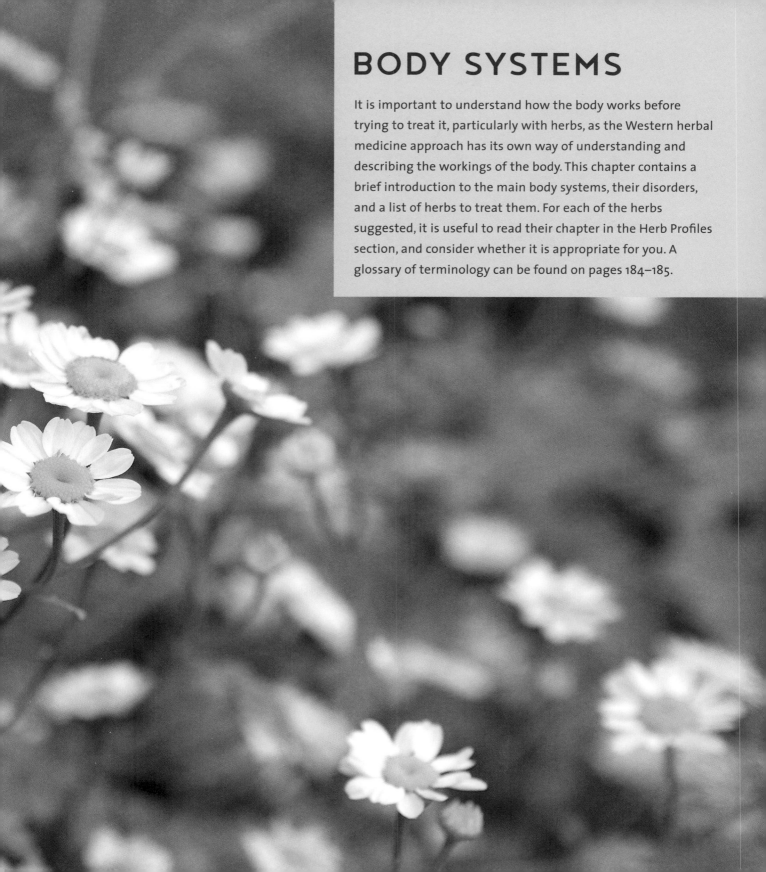

BODY SYSTEMS

It is important to understand how the body works before trying to treat it, particularly with herbs, as the Western herbal medicine approach has its own way of understanding and describing the workings of the body. This chapter contains a brief introduction to the main body systems, their disorders, and a list of herbs to treat them. For each of the herbs suggested, it is useful to read their chapter in the Herb Profiles section, and consider whether it is appropriate for you. A glossary of terminology can be found on pages 184–185.

THE CARDIOVASCULAR SYSTEM

The cardiovascular and circulatory system includes the heart, arteries, and veins. It is an organized pumping system supplying oxygenated blood and nutrients to tissues in the body, and returning deoxygenated blood and waste products back to the liver to filter out toxins and the lungs to be refreshed with oxygen.

The heart and veins are muscular and, like muscles, need to be kept fit and healthy to work efficiently. This is why a diet rich in nutrients, antioxidants, and a balance of healthy fats (particularly omega-3), along with regular moderate exercise, is vital for circulatory health. Some herbs can help to increase the strength of the heartbeat and the efficiency of the system as a whole, and have been used for mild to moderate congestive heart failure. A few of these are incredibly powerful and should only be used under the supervision of a doctor or herbalist due to their potentially toxic nature. Digoxin, a common pharmaceutical drug for heart failure, is derived from the foxglove plant (*Digitalis* spp.).

There are plenty of milder, safer, and effective heart herbs that can improve circulation, reduce cholesterol, and support and strengthen the cardiovascular system. These include hawthorn, linden blossom, and motherwort.

ACTIONS FOR THE CARDIOVASCULAR SYSTEM Circulatory, heart strengthening, vein strengthening, hypotensive, hypertensive, blood pressure balancing, antioxidant.

Hawthorn *Crataegus monogyna* (above).

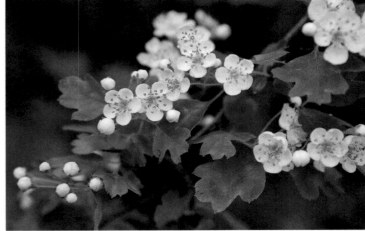

LOVE HEART TEA

This tea is a general circulatory and heart tonic. It is soothing to the nerves and is particularly good for stressed-out people!

- ³/₄ ounce dried hawthorn berries
- ³/₄ ounce dried mixed hawthorn flowers and leaves
- ³/₄ ounce dried linden blossoms
- ³/₄ ounce dried motherwort
- ³/₄ ounce dried mixed yarrow flowers and leaves

Gently crush the hawthorn berries using a mortar and pestle to break them up slightly. Mix with all the other dried herbs in a bowl, then transfer to an airtight container.

To use, add 1–2 teaspoons of the dried herb mixture per cup of boiling water in a mug or teapot. Cover and leave to infuse for 15 minutes. Strain to serve. Alternatively, use an infuser to make the tea.

Take one cup of the tea, up to three times a day.

SHELF LIFE Keep the dried herb mix in a cool, dark place for up to 1 year.

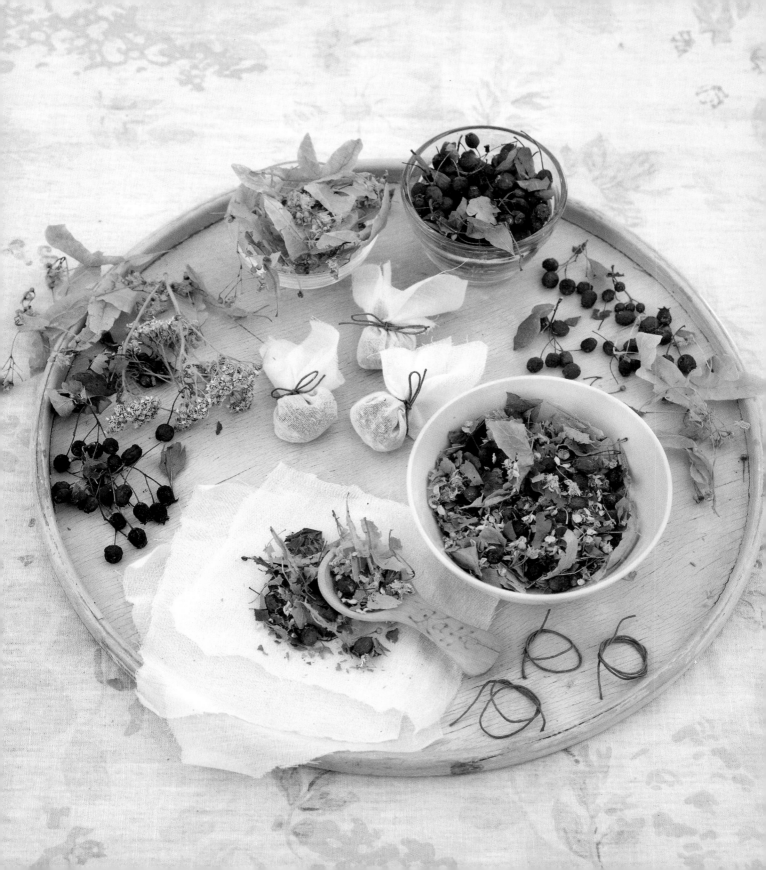

VARICOSE VEINS AND HEMORRHOIDS

Lack of exercise, poor diet, sitting or standing in one position for long periods, and genetic predisposition can all contribute to varicose veins. The vein walls can become stretched and flaccid with blood pooling in the legs, causing knotted-looking veins on the surface of the skin. The legs can feel achy, heavy, and tired, particularly if your day-to-day life is sedentary. Moving the legs around helps tone the muscles that encourage circulation. An effective daily exercise is to lie on your back in a comfortable position, raise your legs in the air, and write the alphabet with your feet.

Hemorrhoids are varicose veins of the rectum.

Both varicose veins and hemorrhoids are worsened by poor digestion and constipation. Make sure you have plenty of fruits and vegetables in your diet for their fiber content and use bitters (see pages 44–45) to help encourage digestion and bowel movements.

Foods and herbs that strengthen the vein walls are also important; antioxidant-rich blue and purple fruits and plants high in the constituent rutin, such as buckwheat and elderflower, should be taken regularly. Horse chestnut and yarrow, used externally, are a simple and effective traditional remedy to encourage circulation and maintain vein wall integrity. Herbs that encourage tissue healing and cool inflammation, such as calendula, St. John's wort, and witch hazel, can also be added to external lotions.

INTERNAL HERBS *Horse Chestnut, Hawthorn, Yarrow, Calendula, St. John's Wort*
EXTERNAL HERBS *Horse Chestnut, Yarrow, Witch Hazel, Calendula, St. John's Wort, Oak bark, Plantain, Selfheal, Rosemary*

VEIN SOOTHING LOTION

This cream is cooling and soothing for varicose veins, spider veins, and hemorrhoids. The astringent properties of witch hazel and oak bark help to shrink the veins, while yarrow and horse chestnut help maintain vein wall integrity.

1 cup aloe vera gel
2 teaspoons horse chestnut leaf–infused oil
2 teaspoons calendula oil
2 teaspoons yarrow tincture
2 teaspoons oak bark tincture
2 teaspoons horse chestnut seed tincture
20 drops of rosemary essential oil (for varicose veins only; omit for hemorrhoids)
2 teaspoons witch hazel

Place the aloe vera gel in a bowl. Slowly add the oils, 1 teaspoon at a time, and whisk thoroughly.

Once combined, add the tinctures, one at a time, and whisk again, then add the essential oil and whisk. Finally, whisk in the witch hazel. Place in a sterilized jar, seal, label, and date.

Alternatively, use a plain base cream instead of the aloe vera gel, and whisk in the oils, tinctures, and witch hazel.

For optimal results, apply this cream twice a day, as well as taking internal circulatory herbs.

SHELF LIFE Up to 1 year in a cool, dark place.

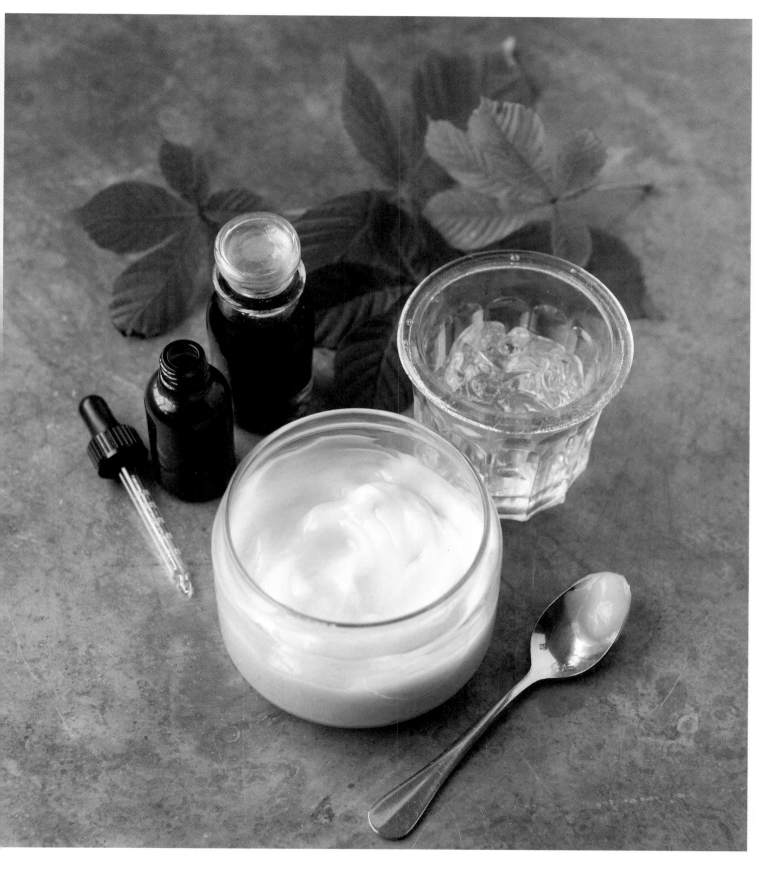

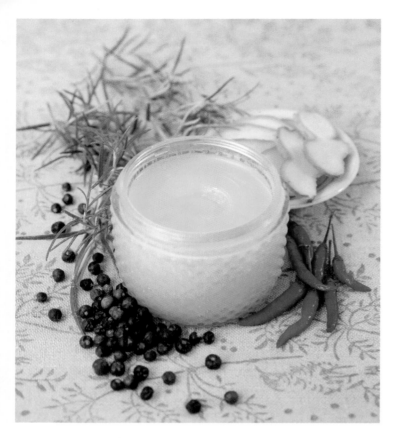

COLD HANDS, FEET, AND CHILBLAINS

In cooler temperatures, blood vessels constrict to reduce blood flow to the extremities to reserve body heat. Some people are more susceptible to temperature shifts and find that they always have cold hands and feet!

Chilblains are painful, itchy blisters that form on the fingers, toes, nose, and ears as a result of fragile blood vessels, due to fluctuations in temperature. If you suffer from cold hands and feet or chilblains, it is important to wear good gloves and socks and try to avoid moving from very cold to hot temperatures. Internal herbal teas using ginger, hawthorn, and yarrow can help improve the circulation and strengthen the veins. Externally, a soothing balm or cream with yarrow and calendula-infused oil can help to heal damaged skin, or try the warming rub below.

INTERNAL HERBS *Yarrow, Elderberry, Elderflower, Hawthorn, Ginger, Chile, Cinnamon, Rosemary*
EXTERNAL HERBS *Calendula, Yarrow, Comfrey, Chile, Ginger, Clove, Juniper, Rosemary*

WARMING RUB

This rub is ideal for cold hands and feet on chilly days. Warming juniper and ginger help assist circulation to the small capillaries in the extremities, while comfrey heals chapped skin.

2 tablespoons chopped fresh rosemary
2 tablespoons dried comfrey leaf
2 tablespoons dried juniper berries, lightly crushed
2-inch piece of fresh ginger, peeled and sliced
1 fresh red chile, chopped
¾ cup olive oil
1 ounce beeswax

Place the herbs, berries, spices, and oil in a bain-marie. Leave to infuse over a very low heat for 2 hours, stirring occasionally.

Strain, discarding the herbs and retaining the oil. Return the oil to the bain-marie, then add the beeswax, stirring until dissolved and melted. Pour into jars, then seal, label, and date.

Apply as needed. Wash hands after applying and do not touch eyes.

SHELF LIFE Up to 2 years.

Yarrow *Alchillea millefolium* (above right).

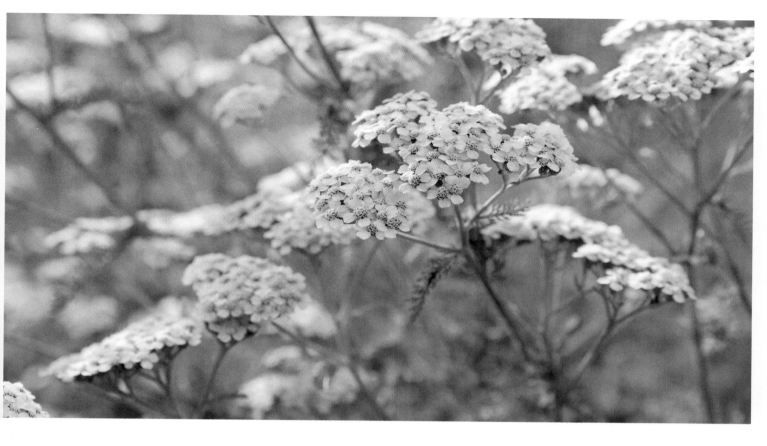

HIGH BLOOD PRESSURE

High blood pressure can be caused by a variety of underlying illnesses, medications, lifestyle, or stress and is a complex subject that should be investigated by a health professional. Untreated it can affect organ function and increases the chance of heart attack and stroke. Regular exercise is essential to maintaining a healthy blood pressure, as is avoiding smoking, excess alcohol, and a diet high in refined fats. Herbal actions for high blood pressure include those that increase the efficacy of the heartbeat, reduce cholesterol, and increase the flexibility of blood vessels. Traditionally, hawthorn is a specific for balancing blood pressure; it works by making the heart pump more efficiently and is often used alone or combined with linden blossom and motherwort as a heart tonic. These herbs also act as anxiolytics, reducing stress and anxiety, one of the main causes of high blood pressure.

HERBS *Hawthorn, Linden blossom, Motherwort, Yarrow, Dandelion, Garlic*

HIGH CHOLESTEROL

Fats are naturally present in our blood, but excess amounts can build up on blood vessel walls leading to restricted blood flow, increased blood pressure, and hardened arteries. Dietary changes are the main approach to treating this condition, i.e. reduce processed meats and junk foods and increase omega-3s, fiber, and antioxidant-rich fruits and vegetables in the diet. Apples, pineapple, nuts, and green tea in particular have been shown to have a positive effect on lowering cholesterol, so try to include these regularly.

Specific herbs that lower cholesterol include those high in antioxidants, such as garlic, ginger, cinnamon, and turmeric, which can be easily incorporated into the diet. Linden blossom has a protective and cholesterol-reducing effect and can be combined with hawthorn, motherwort, and yarrow to act as a general circulatory tonic.

HERBS *Hawthorn, Linden blossom, Birch, Yarrow, Garlic, Yarrow (Achillea millefolium; above), Turmeric, Cinnamon, Ginger*

PALPITATIONS

Palpitations are a noticeable rapid or irregular heartbeat. Most people experience palpitations at some point in their lives. They can be caused by a variety of issues from anxiety to thyroid conditions, but if they are recurring or cause light-headedness, you should get checked over by a doctor to rule out other issues. Palpitations from anxiety can be eased with the following herbs that help soothe stress and support heart function.

HERBS *Hawthorn, Linden blossom, Motherwort, Yarrow, Lemon Balm, Skullcap*

ANEMIA

Simple iron-deficiency anemia can cause tiredness, pallor, and dizziness and, if it's not treated, can lead to further health problems. Identify the underlying cause: is it due to poor diet, inefficient absorption of minerals from the diet, or heavy menstrual bleeding? Increase iron-rich foods in the diet with dark green leafy vegetables, sunflower seeds, red meat, or tofu. Digestive stimulants, such as bitters, increase digestive juices that in turn increase mineral absorption.

For anemia caused by heavy menstrual bleeding, see the Female Reproductive System section on page 50 for herbs that balance the hormones and reduce menstrual flow.

Nettles are mineral rich, particularly in iron, and are classed as a traditional blood tonic. They can be taken in strong infusions but are particularly nourishing when juiced or eaten. Try the Nettle Tonic recipe on the right.

HERBS *Nettles, Curly Dock, Burdock, Raspberry leaf, Horsetail, Dandelion leaf*

NETTLE TONIC

This recipe makes a tasty tonic wine that can be used as a general tonic or for treating iron-deficiency anemia. If you would like to make a more traditional tonic wine, you can add curly dock root—however, this makes it quite bitter!

2 handfuls of nettle tops
a handful of raspberry leaves
a handful of dandelion leaves
2 handfuls of sulfur-free dried apricots
2 tablespoons curly dock root (optional)
peel from 1 orange or lemon
     (organic and unwaxed), cut into strips
1 bottle (750 ml) red wine
2 tablespoons molasses
½ cup brandy

Finely chop the herbs and dried apricots and place in large sterilized jars. Add the dock root (if using) and orange or lemon peel. Cover with the red wine, molasses, and brandy. Seal the jar and leave to infuse for 2 weeks in a cool, dark place, shaking occasionally.

Strain into a clean sterilized jar, pressing the liquid from the herbs, then seal, label, and date. Keep in the fridge.

Take 2 tablespoons with meals, as needed.

SHELF LIFE Up to 2 months in the fridge (discard if it smells vinegary).

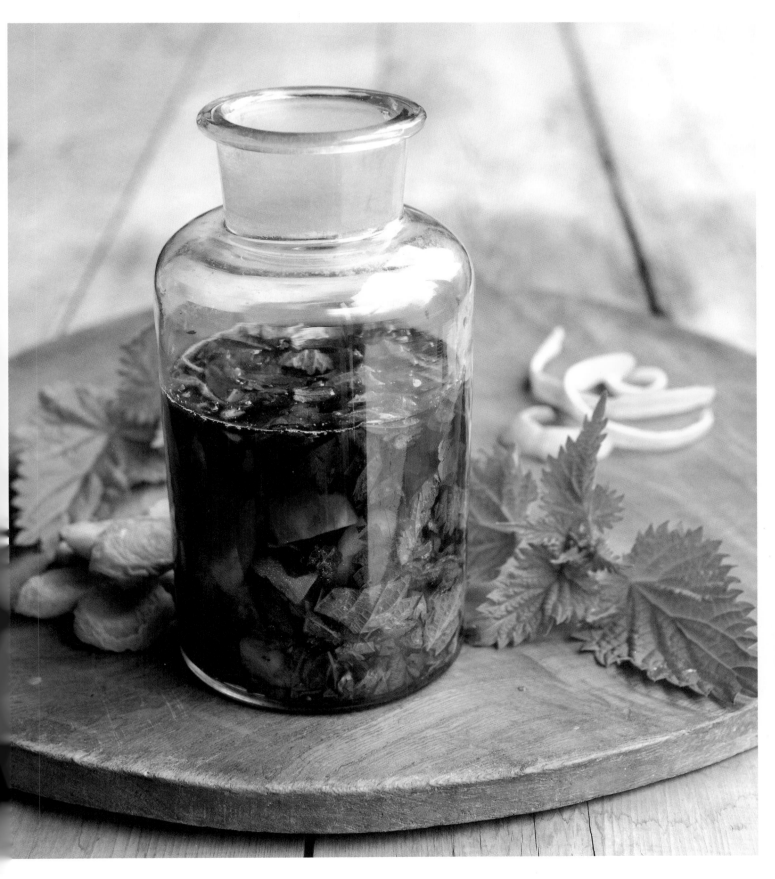

THE DIGESTIVE SYSTEM

Good health starts with good food and good digestion. How our bodies use the nutrients we consume is essential to our overall state of health. If the digestive system is not working efficiently, our bodies cannot capture the nutrients that produce the building blocks and energy we need for vital bodily functions including growth, repair and hormone messengers.

There is a fine line between food and medicine. Many of the culinary herbs we use are aromatic or bitter for good reason. These tastes can benefit digestion through various actions, including stimulating, relaxing, or antimicrobial effects. The modern diet is high in sweet and salty flavors but lacking in bitter foods, and this unbalanced combination can make for a sluggish digestive system that can affect our vitality and the rest of the body. Adding bitter foods and herbs to the diet stimulates the liver and the first stages of digestion (see Liver and Bitters, right).

Around 70 percent of our immune tissue is located in the digestive tract, meaning that gut health is imperative to overall health. Poor digestive health can cause reactions to food and chronic inflammation, making the body more prone to infections, allergies and a whole host of other illnesses. Healing, soothing mucilaginous herbs, as well as astringent, tannin-rich herbs and bitters, can help tone up an inflamed digestive tract.

We have a symbiotic relationship with the colony of bacteria living within our gut and what we put into our body affects what gut flora we "cultivate". Simply put, "friendly" bacteria flourish with wholesome foods, whereas "unfriendly" bacteria prefer sugary, fatty foods. It's a fact that these bacterial cells outnumber our own cells—they're just much smaller.

So cultivate your bacterial friends and help them stay healthy, particularly after illness or a course of antibiotics. Eat a diet low in refined sugars and high in a wide range of fruits and vegetables. Add fermented foods such as kimchi (see page 27), yogurt, sauerkraut, and traditionally made miso, along with bitter herbs and roots that either contain the "good" bacteria (probiotics) or substances they thrive on (prebiotics).

Ever had a "gut feeling"? New research shows that the type of gut flora you have may be associated with mood, anxiety, and certain diseases. If stress plays a role in your digestive disturbance, nervine and adaptogenic herbs can help your body cope and reduce these symptoms.

For chronic and recurring problems, particularly with the suspicion of food intolerances, keeping a food and symptoms diary can be useful. It can help you establish links between symptoms, your diet, and life events. Try an elimination diet: cut out suspect foods (for example, wheat or dairy) for at least two months before reintroducing them a tiny bit at a time. Note down any reactions in a journal.

ACTIONS FOR THE DIGESTIVE SYSTEM Demulcent, anti-inflammatory, astringent, carminative, bitter, hepatic, antimicrobial, laxative, relaxant, nervine, antispasmodic.

THE LIVER AND BITTERS

There are bitter receptors all around our bodies; in the mouth, digestive tract, and even the skin. Bitter herbs stimulate the digestion, enzyme production, bile, and gastric juices to enable nutrients to be broken down and absorbed more efficiently.

The liver produces bile to neutralize stomach acid, break down food, and act as a laxative. It is the body's natural detoxification center; it processes wastes and eliminates excess hormones and toxins from the body. Bitters support liver function and are helpful in many conditions, particularly hormonal issues, skin problems, immune function, and allergies.

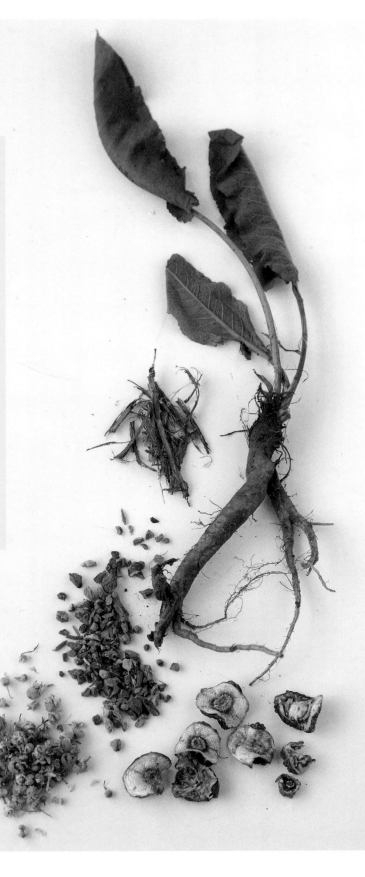

BITTER HERBS

Angelica root (*Angelica archangelica*)
Burdock root (*Arctium lappa*)
Berberis bark (*Berberis aquifolium*)
Chicory root (*Cichorium intybus*)
Chamomile flower (*Matricaria chamomilla*)
Curly or Curled Dock (*Rumex crispus*)
Dandelion (*Taraxacum officinale*)

BITTER DIGESTIVE DROPS

Chop and place a mixture of any of the above herbs with some chopped orange peel in a sterilized preserving jar and fully cover with vodka (see Tinctures on page 15). Leave in a cool, dark place and gently shake every few days. After a month, strain and pour the liquid into a sterilized dropper bottle. Seal, label, and date. Take 10–20 drops in 2 tablespoons of water, 15–30 minutes before meals, as needed.

CAUTIONS People with gastric ulcers should see an herbalist before trying bitters. Do not use in pregnancy.

MOUTH ULCERS

Mouth ulcers are painful sores that can appear on the gums, tongue, and inner cheeks. They usually occur during times of stress or illness. Use vulnerary herbs like calendula to heal tissues, along with antimicrobial and astringent herbs such as sage, raspberry leaf, or eucalyptus. Try swilling your mouth with a strong infusion of calendula petals or brew up the Mouthwash recipe on page 107.

BAD BREATH

Ruling out poor oral hygiene, deeper digestive unhappiness may be the cause for smelly breath. Sluggish digestion, perhaps due to low stomach acid, can cause food to sit in the gut for long periods, resulting in unpleasant gases and odors. Use bitter herbs (see Liver and Bitters on page 44) to stimulate digestion, and aromatic herbs, such as fennel, parsley, and mint, after meals to sweeten the breath. The Healing Ulcer Mouthwash on page 107 will also help improve oral hygiene.

HERBS *Parsley, Fennel, Dandelion root, Curly Dock, Burdock, Mint, Sage*

HEARTBURN

That burning, uncomfortable feeling in the center of your chest after eating food is often blamed on excess stomach acid. In fact, heartburn can also be caused by a low stomach acid, or a weak sphincter at the top of the stomach allowing the regurgitation of acid into the gullet.

Antacids suppress the production of stomach acid, relieving symptoms of heartburn short-term but often worsen it in the long run. Suppressing stomach acid can prevent proper digestion and even cause the stomach to reflexively produce more acid. Instead, try soothing and gently stimulating bitter herbs before or after a meal, such as the Bitter Digestive Drops (see box on page 45) or a traditional chamomile and meadowsweet infusion.

Peppermint should be avoided as it relaxes the top of the stomach, which allows acid to creep up and may worsen the symptoms. If you have a gastric ulcer, consult an herbalist before treating with herbs, particularly bitters.

HERBS *Chamomile, Meadowsweet, Dandelion, Angelica, Oats, Marshmallow, Slippery Elm, Calendula*

NAUSEA

Nausea after eating can be caused by food intolerances or low stomach acid. Bitters again will help stimulate and settle the stomach. Fresh ginger root infusions are invaluable here and this herb is also helpful in morning and motion sickness. Chronic nausea should be checked out by a health professional.

HERBS *Ginger, Chamomile, Dandelion root, Fennel, Meadowsweet*

STOMACHACHES

Stomachaches may be caused by the discomfort of trapped wind (see Flatulence and Bloating on page 47). Acute, sudden pain or pain that recurs over time may need the attention of a medical professional. Peppermint tea can help digestive discomfort.

HEMORRHOIDS

Hemorrhoids are varicose veins of the rectum. See Varicose Veins in the Cardiovascular section on page 38.

INFLAMMATORY BOWEL DISEASE (IBD) AND OTHER CHRONIC DIGESTIVE DISORDERS

Inflammatory bowel disease (a term usually used to describe two conditions, ulcerative colitis and Crohn's disease), irritable bowel syndrome (IBS), and celiac disease are all complex, uncomfortable, and disruptive conditions. The symptomatic relief of wind, diarrhea, and constipation at home with herbs may be helpful, but do seek assistance with an herbalist for a more holistic approach, particularly if you are on any medications.

FLATULENCE AND BLOATING

Wind (up or down) can be caused by a variety of factors including eating too fast, poor stomach acid, gut bacteria imbalance, and food insensitivities. Pay attention to posture and speed when eating; take your time and chew food thoroughly—you might find this simple action really helps!

An imbalance of gut bacteria can cause food to ferment in the digestive tract and produce gas as a by-product. Think of how certain bacteria make fermented drinks, such as champagne, fizzy! Trapped wind can cause a lot of discomfort as pressure builds up. Aromatic carminative herbs such as fennel, angelica, and peppermint can help to reduce spasm and the buildup of gas.

HERBS *Fennel seed, Dill, Chamomile, Mint, Ginger, Dandelion Root, Angelica, Parsley, Peppermint*

CONSTIPATION

Different people generally have different bowel habits, but it is important to establish what is normal for you. Generally, at least one bowel movement a day is ideal. Check out the Bristol Stool Chart online, which can help you assess healthy bowel movements, making you aware of any changes.

Constipation can be caused by diets low in fiber, or it can be a side effect from certain medications or illness. It can also happen when people feel tense and "clench up." In this case, relaxing nervine herbs such as vervain or chamomile are best. It is important to drink lots of water, which acts as a lubricant for the gut. If you don't drink enough, your body will try to reabsorb it before you go to the toilet, causing hard stools that are difficult to pass.

Irritant laxatives, such as senna or cascara, are sometimes used for constipation, but these can be harsh—they irritate the gut, causing expulsion. If used frequently, the body can become reliant on them and may find it hard to "go" without them. These herbs should be used sparingly in rare situations and never constantly. Instead, stimulate proper digestion with bitters before eating and use bulk laxatives; gentle demulcent herbs that help the stools to retain more water, softening and lubricating the bowels.

Demulcent herbs include psyllium husks, slippery elm, marshmallow root, and even oats—they contain "gloopy" mucilages that hold water and make things "slippery." Use them as powders—add to cold water and allow them to sit until they are gloopy and then drink them down. If you take medications, it is best to leave 45 minutes before taking them, as they are so good at coating the gut, they may prevent absorption.

HERBS *Oats, Slippery Elm, Marshmallow root, Psyllium husk, Dandelion root, Burdock, Curly Dock, Berberis*

DIARRHEA

Diarrhea is the body's way of clearing unwanted substances, including microbes in the gut, so suppressing diarrhea is not always desirable, as it can cause infection to remain in the system. During bouts of diarrhea, drink plenty of fluids. Rehydration salts can be made at home using 7 level teaspoons of sugar and 1 level teaspoon of salt to 1 quart water, and the juice of an orange. If the diarrhea is severe or prolonged, particularly in the case of children or the elderly, professional help must be sought.

Herbal treatments for diarrhea include antimicrobials for infection control (such as in food poisoning). Astringent herbs should be taken to tone the intestinal mucous membranes and prevent further loss of liquids. Use strong herbal infusions for the added bonus of getting liquids and minerals back into the body.

Roman chamomile (Chamaemelum nobile) is an excellent treatment as part of any herbal mix, helping calm griping pains as well as being powerfully antimicrobial. After an illness such as norovirus, boost the immune system for a swifter recovery and rebuild the gut lining with a soothing Chicken Bone Broth (see recipe on page 56).

HERBS *Chamomile, Thyme, Sage, Oregano, Berberis, Licorice, Oak bark, Meadowsweet, Echinacea, Blackberry leaf, Raspberry leaf*

CHEWABLE IMMUNE-GUT GUMMIES

These gummies contain tasty, immune-boosting, antimicrobial elderberry and thyme and gut-soothing licorice. They are ideal for tummies recovering from illness, where the gelatin or agar-agar will help to coat and soothe the digestive tract, heal the gut lining, and relieve constipation. This remedy also doubles up as a treatment for colds, flu, sore throats, and coughs. The gummy form makes them a success for fussy children.

3 tablespoons (1¾ ounces) fresh elderberries
1 teaspoon chopped or powdered licorice root
1 star anise (optional)
1 cinnamon stick (optional)
1 tablespoon chopped fresh thyme
1 tablespoon honey
4 tablespoons gelatin granules/powder OR
    2 tablespoons agar-agar flakes (vegan option)

Place the elderberries, licorice, and spices (if using) in a small saucepan with ¾ cup water. Bring to a boil, then reduce the heat, cover, and simmer gently for 10 minutes.

Remove from the heat, stir in the thyme, cover again, and leave for another 5 minutes.

Strain the liquid through a strainer, pushing the berries through. Discard the seeds, thyme, spices, and any licorice root left in the strainer.

Stir the honey into the strained liquid until dissolved. Measure the liquid. It should now be approximately ¾ cup of liquid. If it is not, then top up with a little hot water.

If using gelatin, sprinkle the gelatin over the hot liquid and whisk thoroughly until completely dissolved. Scoop off any froth and discard. Pour the mixture into silicone molds (we use silicone chocolatier molds; see also Tip), then place in the fridge for up to 1 hour until set. To remove the gummies from the silicone molds, you may need to sit the base of the mold in warm water for 5–10 minutes (this softens the gummies slightly to release them); they should then pop out easily.

If using agar-agar flakes, leave the liquid to cool, then return it to the pan. Sprinkle the flakes over the liquid and then bring to a boil, without stirring. Reduce the heat and simmer until the flakes are completely dissolved, stirring occasionally, about 10–15 minutes. Pour the mix into silicone molds (or see Tip), then leave to set in the fridge—setting will happen very quickly, about 20 minutes max. Once set, these should easily pop out of the molds.

Store in an airtight container in the fridge for up to a week. They can be frozen for up to 6 months, but turn mushy, so stir them into hot water for a soothing drink.

To use, take one as needed, up to four times a day.

TIP If you don't have a silicone chocolatier's mold, pour the mixture into a plastic wrap–lined small baking sheet or shallow glass dish and leave to set in the fridge, then cut into small cubes.

SHELF LIFE Up to 1 week in the fridge.

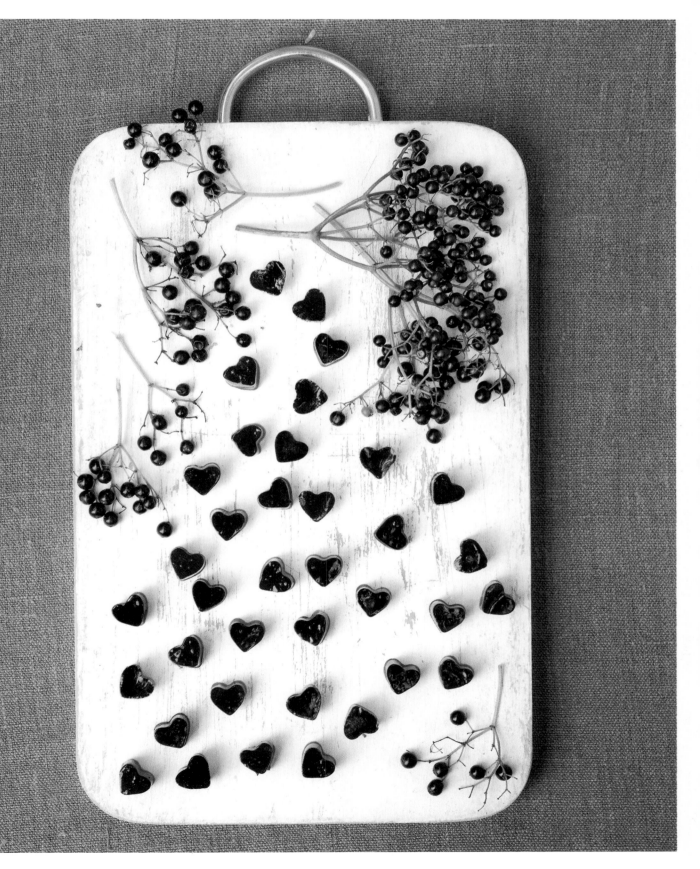

THE FEMALE REPRODUCTIVE SYSTEM

The female reproductive system is a truly remarkable thing, governed by complex and delicately balanced hormonal exchanges. Many diseases of the female system arise from an imbalance of the two major reproductive hormones, estrogen and progesterone.

Our reproductive system is very much affected by our overall health. The fragile ebb and flow of hormones that keep a woman's cycle in balance are easily affected by stress, diet, and general lifestyle. Mainstream medicine tends to focus on the reduction of symptoms, using painkillers and hormonal-based medicines. While these can be helpful, they rarely treat the root of the problem.

Herbal treatment for the female system focuses on identifying imbalance, using herbs that work synergistically with the body to help level out hormones and improve symptoms. Nourishing herbs for the nervous and endocrine systems, such as licorice and skullcap, can help relieve hormonal imbalance associated with stress, while liver clearing and bitter herbs help clear excess hormones from the body by filtering them from the blood. From menstrual problems such as premenstrual syndrome (PMS) and painful periods, to menopausal hot flashes, herbs have a wonderful host of healing potential at any stage of life.

Chronic complications such as endometriosis, infertility, polycystic ovary disease, and fibroids can be positively approached with herbs and dietary changes, but due to their complicated nature, it is best to seek advice from a medical practitioner or herbalist.

Unexplained sudden changes in your cycle, such as increased or irregular bleeding, require professional medical treatment and diagnosis.

CAUTION Always consult with a qualified medical herbalist while trying to conceive or when pregnant.

KEEPING TRACK

There is no such thing as a "one size fits all" cycle; every woman has a cycle that is unique to her, but knowing what is normal for you is important. Keeping a menstrual diary can be a powerful tool; it helps you to be in tune with your cycle and fertility and pinpoint any irregularities. To keep a menstrual diary, note the first to the last day of bleeding and record the quality of blood, e.g. heavy, light, red, dark, clots. Take note of any other symptoms before, during, and after your period too; skin condition, emotions, breast tenderness, libido changes. There are many free apps that can help with this.

ACTIONS FOR THE FEMALE REPRODUCTIVE SYSTEM
Uterine tonic, emmenagogue, hormone regulator, nutritive, alterative, pelvic decongestant, circulatory, adaptogen.

HEAVY PERIODS

Heavy periods can be an indicator of other underlying problems, such as fibroids or endometriosis, but for many women they are part of their "normal" monthly cycle and are simply uncomfortable. Uterine astringent herbs work to tighten the tissues of the womb and lessen bleeding; these include raspberry leaf, lady's mantle, and yarrow.

The best way to reap the tonifying effects of these herbs is to take them as an infusion or tincture regularly throughout the month. One of the most powerful uterine astringents is shepherd's purse; take it daily for 7–10 days before and during the period to lessen heavy bleeding. If you do bleed heavily every month, nutritive herbs like nettle can help to replenish lost minerals; see the Nettle Tonic recipe on page 42.

HERBS *Raspberry leaf, Lady's Mantle, Yarrow, Shepherd's Purse, Self-heal*

WOMEN'S BALANCE TEA

This tea combines hormone-balancing rose and lady's mantle with adaptogenic nervines, skullcap and licorice. It can be drunk throughout the month to relieve premenstrual tension and help regulate the cycles.

1 ounce dried rose
1 ounce dried lady's mantle
1 ounce dried skullcap
½ ounce licorice powder (optional)

Mix all the dried herbs and licorice powder (if using) together and keep in an airtight container.

Place 1–2 teaspoons of the dried herb mix in 1 cup of boiling water, cover, and steep for 15 minutes. Strain and drink. Drink up to three times a day.

SHELF LIFE Keep the dried herb mix in a cool, dark place for up to 1 year.

TEA FOR HEAVY MENSTRUAL BLEEDING

This tea can be drunk throughout the month or just for the week preceding the period to lessen heavy bleeding.

1 ounce dried lady's mantle
1 ounce dried raspberry leaf
1 ounce dried yarrow
1 ounce dried self-heal
1 ounce dried nettle leaf

Mix all the dried herbs together and keep in an airtight container.

Place 1–2 teaspoons of the dried herb mix in 1 cup of boiling water, cover, and steep for 15 minutes. Strain and drink. Drink up to three times a day.

SHELF LIFE Keep the dried herb mix in a cool, dark place for up to 1 year.

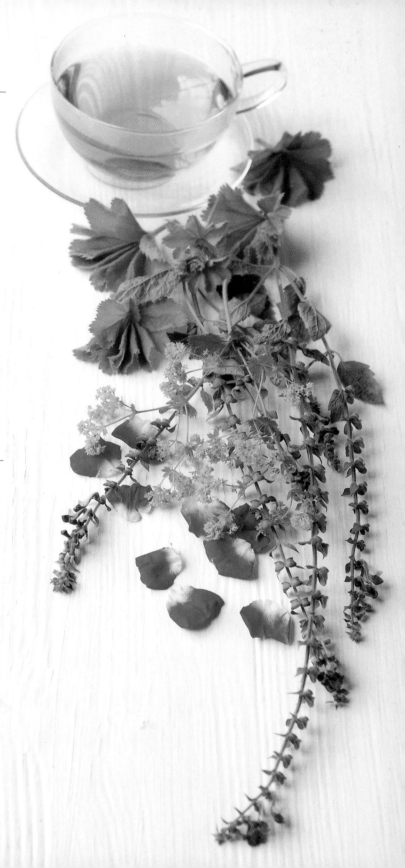

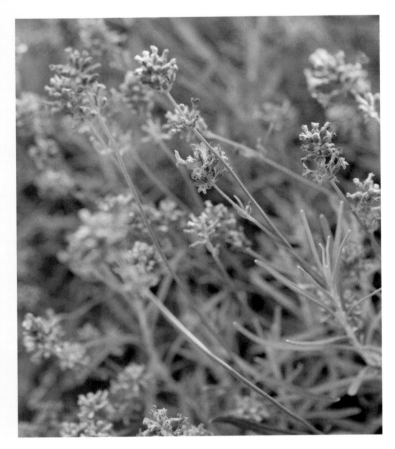

THRUSH

The vagina is a delicate ecosystem full of naturally occurring bacteria and fungi, much like the gut. Thrush is caused by an imbalance of vaginal flora, usually by an overgrowth of candida, a fungus that is normally present in the vagina, leading to inflammation and discomfort.

Stress, tight clothing, poor gut health, antibiotics, and hormonal birth control drugs can all alter the balance of flora in the vagina. Eating a diet high in prebiotic and probiotic foods, such as fresh garlic, live yogurt, and fermented vegetables, can help re-establish a healthy balance of flora. An Herbal Sitz Bath (see page 85 in the Urinary section) can help to relieve itchiness and soothe irritation.

HERBS *Lavender, Calendula, Thyme, Echinacea, Lady's Mantle, Oregano, Eucalyptus*

Lavender *Lavandula angustifolia* (above)

MENOPAUSAL SYMPTOMS

For some women, menopause passes by with little more than hot flashes. For others it can be a time of upheaval, both emotionally and physically. Regardless of experience, menopause is a time of great change within the body and a time where a bit of holistic herbal support can work wonders.

The symptoms of menopause are largely caused by falling levels of various hormones, particularly estrogen. Phytoestrogens are plant-based compounds that can mildly mimic estrogen, reducing the symptoms of menopause, such as hot flashes and vaginal dryness.

Consuming a varied diet high in whole foods and vegetables can dramatically improve the severity of menopausal symptoms. Phytoestrogen-containing foods include organic fermented soy products, such as miso, tempeh and tofu, as well as pulses, grains, vegetables, and seeds (specifically flax and sesame seeds). Many herbs contain phytoestrogens too, so use lots of fresh culinary herbs in cooking to benefit from them, or drink daily herbal infusions. Some well-known phytoestrogen-containing herbs include sage and red clover.

Erratic cycles leading up to menopause are common, with menstruation occurring more or less frequently than usual. Some women also experience flooding, or very heavy bleeding, which can lead to anemia, in which case, use the same herbs as described in the Heavy Periods section on page 50.

Hot flashes can be embarrassing and uncomfortable and can affect sleeping patterns too. Sage is the traditional remedy for hot flashes, as are lemon balm and elderflower; these are herbs that have a diaphoretic effect and are usually used for fever, as they encourage the body's natural cooling processes.

During menopause, hormone levels can fluctuate massively in a way not too dissimilar from when periods are first being established during the teen years. Symptoms often resemble PMS, in which case, treat with the appropriate remedies for PMS (see section opposite).

The hormonal disruption can have psychological and emotional effects with many women experiencing low mood, anxiety, and forgetfulness. This tends to settle down once periods have come to a complete stop but can be helped along with anxiolytic herbs such as St. John's wort, rose, skullcap, lemon balm, and linden blossom.

Falling levels of estrogen can cause a significant drop in bone density, leading to bone fractures and osteoporosis (porous bones). Osteoporosis and low bone mass is thought to affect up to 50 percent of postmenopausal women (aged 50–80 years). A number of studies have shown that women who take up exercise before menopause starts experience less severe menopausal symptoms in general (also see the Osteoporosis section on page 61). Overnight infusions of nettle, plantain, horsetail, raspberry leaf, and other mineral-rich herbs taken daily are a great way to boost vital bone nutrients, without the need for "supercharged," super expensive nutritional supplements.

CAUTION If bleeding occurs more than one year after having no periods, contact your medical practitioner.

HERBS *Red Clover, Nettle, Plantain, Raspberry leaf, Sage, Shepherd's Purse, Yarrow, Lemon Balm, Rose, Elderflower, St. John's Wort, Skullcap, Linden blossom, Lady's Mantle, Self-heal*

PAINFUL PERIODS

Painful periods are usually caused by an imbalance of naturally occurring bodily chemicals and hormones. The main group of chemicals responsible for pain are prostaglandins; these are hormone-like substances that help the body when it's injured by causing blood to rush to the area. In the womb, prostaglandins help with muscle contractions that discard the uterine lining but can also cause inflammation, resulting in cramping and pain. Most over-the-counter painkillers are anti-inflammatory and reduce pain by preventing the body from producing too many prostaglandins. Many herbs act in this anti-inflammatory way too.

Weak muscles in the uterus also contribute to pain

and spasm; traditional women's herbs, such as lady's mantle and raspberry leaf, help to tone and strengthen the uterus. Antispasmodic herbs like crampbark, fennel, and chamomile can reduce pain from muscle spasm. "Stagnation" of blood is often described in traditional Chinese medicine (TCM) as a cause for painful periods, so add some circulation-stimulating herbs, such as yarrow and ginger, to a soothing infusion to encourage the movement of blood and enhance the actions of other herbs.

HERBS *Lady's Mantle, Crampbark, Meadowsweet, Calendula, Chamomile, Yarrow, Ginger, Poppy, Juniper*

PREMENSTRUAL SYNDROME (PMS)

PMS tends to be caused by fluctuating hormone levels just before menstruation. Symptoms are variable and are specific to the individual, but commonly include sugar cravings, bloating, irritability, lack of concentration, fatigue, and breast tenderness. Dietary deficiencies can contribute massively, and many women find supplementing with magnesium, B vitamins, and essential fatty acids beneficial. As symptoms are so varied, treatment plans with a range of herbal actions should be tailored to individual needs.

Bitter herbs aid in the removal of excess hormones by stimulating the liver and helping it to detoxify the system. Diuretic herbs, like dandelion leaf, help to lessen bloating and water retention. Anxiolytic herbs can soften mood swings and reduce emotional tension. Motherwort and lady's mantle are good all-rounders, as they gently balance the hormones and tone the reproductive system as a whole.

A highly effective herb for normalizing hormones is chasteberry (Vitex agnus-castus), and is well worth investigating if you are a PMS sufferer. However, the dosage is very specific to the individual, so it is best to consult an herbalist to find out what amount is suitable for you before trying it.

HERBS *Dandelion leaf, Motherwort, Lady's Mantle, Chasteberry, St. John's Wort, Skullcap, Vervain, Angelica, Cleavers*

THE IMMUNE SYSTEM

The immune system is the body's defense against illness and infection. It isn't one specific organ or tissue but involves the interplay between bone marrow, an army of white blood cells, the lymphatic system, spleen, certain glands, and even your digestive flora. Overall, it has the ability to recognize, regulate, and remove anything that has the potential to infect or damage the body, including bacteria, viruses, and mutated cells.

The immune system is incredibly complex and usually works without us even noticing, but we do tend to notice when it becomes out of balance. We do not just "catch" infections; they usually occur when we stop listening to our body's warning signs: when we are overworked, stressed, and eating unhealthily we provide the right environment for infection to thrive.

To keep the immune system running smoothly, make sure your body is well equipped to combat infection: research shows that a healthy diet, regular exercise, and taking care to manage stress levels all have positive effects on the immune system. However, no matter how healthy the lifestyle, everyone is open to illness from time to time. In these cases, herbs provide extra support to allow the body to heal itself.

Prevention, they say, is better than cure, and there are many herbs that are used to enhance the immune system. Some are used as general tonics to boost overall vitality and others are used at the first sign of infection. One of the top antimicrobial herbs used in herbal medicine is garlic. Research trials show that people with diets higher in garlic suffer from fewer cold and flu infections, so eat more garlic!

When the immune system is in a state of disorder, it can be looked at in two ways: it can be underactive, causing you to seemingly pick up every infection going, or it can be overactive, triggering a range of allergy-like symptoms, such as hay fever or some autoimmune disorders.

For underactive immune systems, increase your body's ability to fight infection. Echinacea and elderberry enhance the production of white blood cells, which engulf and destroy foreign bodies such as bacteria and viruses.

For overreactive immune systems, aim to "normalize" the immune response with alteratives and adaptogens that balance function.

For specific infections, see the information on specific body systems; e.g. for cystitis, see the Urinary section on pages 84–85.

ACTIONS FOR THE IMMUNE SYSTEM Alterative, adaptogen, antiviral, antibacterial, antifungal, immune-enhancing.

ALTERATIVES AND ADAPTOGENS

Adaptogens are nature's balancers. They amplify the body's resilience to infection and help maintain equilibrium. They are particularly used in herbal medicine for treating both stress and the immune system (for more on adaptogens for stress, see page 67).

Traditionally, alteratives were known as "blood cleansers". They act to gradually "alter" a diseased body back into a state of balance, through cleansing the blood and encouraging the breakdown and elimination of metabolic waste in an overburdened system. Some herbs can be both adaptogens and alteratives and the difference between the two can be blurred.

Mushrooms, such as shiitake and birch polypore, are used for deep immune system balancing, so it's a good idea to include a range of different mushrooms in the diet. Shiitake and wild mushrooms can be purchased from most supermarkets and are rich in immune-enhancing constituents, including various polysaccharides, particularly ß-glucans.

HERBS *Licorice, Echinacea, Nettle, Burdock, Cleavers, Shiitake and Birch Polypore Mushrooms*

HERBAL HAND SANITIZER

Prevention is better than cure. This natural hand sanitizer combines antimicrobial herbs to kill the bugs that cause infection. It can be used when out and about without the need for water.

¼ cup aloe vera gel
2 teaspoons herbal-infused oil
1 teaspoon thyme tincture
10 drops of lavender essential oil
10 drops of eucalyptus essential oil

Put the aloe vera gel into a small mixing bowl, then slowly add the infused oil, whisking together thoroughly. Add the tincture and essential oils and whisk again.

Pour into pump or squeeze bottles, seal, label, and date. Use as needed.

SHELF LIFE Up to 1 year in a cool, dark place.

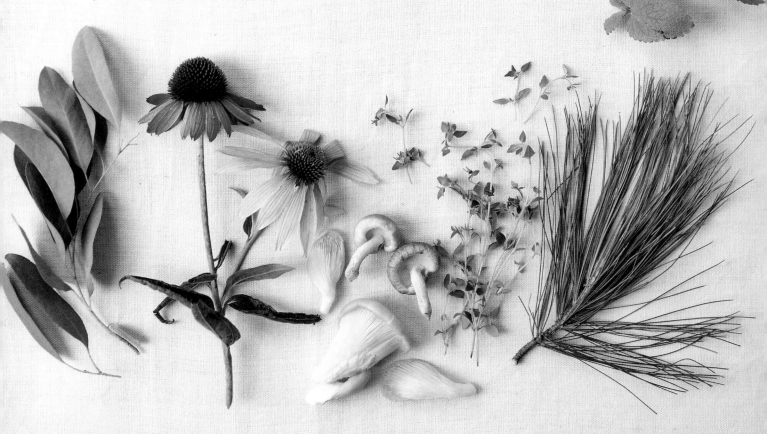

CHICKEN BONE BROTH

Chicken soup is a powerful kitchen remedy, beneficial to almost any ailment. It contains a wide range of bioavailable proteins, nutrients, and minerals, such as arginine, glutamine, calcium, magnesium, phosphorus, silicon, sulfur chondroitin, and glucosamine. It boosts collagen production for healthy joints, skin, and membranes, and is particularly beneficial for gut health and rebuilding the intestinal lining after vomiting or digestive upsets.

1 large onion
2 carrots, peeled
3 celery stalks
4 garlic cloves
1 raw or cooked (roasted) organic chicken carcass (or use 10–15 organic chicken wings)
2 handfuls of fresh nettles (or a handful of dried)
a handful of fresh thyme
4 bay leaves

Roughly chop the vegetables and garlic. Place them in a large saucepan with the chicken carcass and herbs, then pour in 2 quarts of water. Bring to a boil, then reduce the heat, cover, and simmer gently for 3–4 hours. Keep an eye on the water level, topping it up if needed, and if any foam appears, skim it off and discard.

Once cooked, strain the broth, discarding the solids, then drink/serve the broth as it is in a mug or bowl, or use it as stock for soups, risotto, sauces, and gravies.

Alternatively, strain the broth, remove the chicken bones, nettles, thyme stalks, and bay leaves, then return the vegetables and broth to the pan. Blend (using a stick blender in the pan) until smooth to serve as a soup, adding stock or water to achieve the right consistency, then reheat before serving. For an added collagen boost, garnish with the Rosehip Powder on page 133.

SHELF LIFE This broth will keep in an airtight container in the fridge for up to 3 days, or it can be frozen for up to 3 months (defrost overnight in the fridge before use).

VEGAN VERSION Instead of chicken, use 2 quarts of water with 1 strip of kombu and 1 ounce wakame seaweed (both easily purchased from many supermarkets in the Asian section), 3½ ounces shiitake mushrooms, and 1¾ ounces whole rosehips, and simmer together gently for 1–2 hours. Remove the kombu and rosehips before serving.

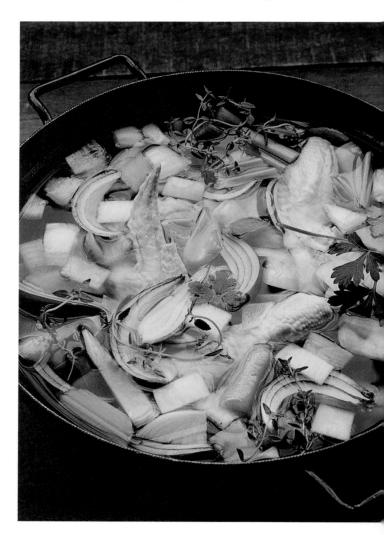

BACTERIAL INFECTIONS

Herbs produce naturally occurring, antibacterial chemicals to protect themselves from disease. Culinary herbs are particularly effective antibacterials, and this is one of the reasons they are used in cooking—as well as tasting good, their essential oils help to preserve food. The antibacterial actions of these aromatic herbs can be used internally for bacterial infections including stomach upsets and respiratory and urinary infections. They are also effective externally in creams and balms for small, infected cuts and wounds.

HERBS *Thyme, Rosemary, Sage, Oregano, Eucalyptus, Calendula, Lavender, Melissa, Self-heal, Plantain, Garlic, Cinnamon, Basil, Ginger, Juniper, Echinacea*

VIRAL INFECTIONS

Viruses are small particles that use the body's own cells to replicate, destroying them in the process. Antibiotics do not work on viruses and should be avoided unless there is a secondary bacterial infection. Powerful antiviral herbs, such as elderberry and thyme, act in a variety of ways, including preventing viruses from attaching to cell walls and replicating.

HERBS *Elderberry, Elderflower, Echinacea, Eucalyptus, St. John's Wort, Lemon Balm, Thyme*

FUNGAL INFECTIONS

We all have naturally occurring "friendly" fungi that live in our bodies. Fungal infections usually occur when the immune system is compromised, allowing either our native fungi to become overgrown, or invading fungi to cause infection. Fungal infections are particularly at home in warm, dark, damp places, such as the feet and groin, leading to conditions such as athlete's foot, thrush, and ringworm. When treating fungal infections, treat the immune system with herbs such as echinacea and elderberry, along with topical antifungal herbs.

HERBS *Oregano, Thyme, Eucalyptus, Calendula, Echinacea, Elderberry*

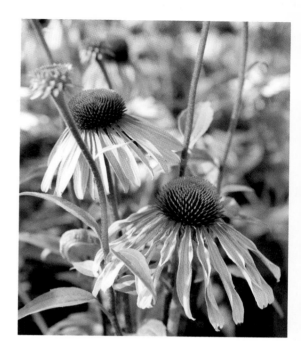

IMMUNE TONIC TINCTURE

Echinacea and elderberry are two herbs used to boost the immune system for prevention and treatment of infection. Combine the health-enhancing effects of mushrooms and antimicrobial properties of eucalyptus and you have an all-round infection-busting tonic.

7 ounces fresh elderberries (or 3½ ounces dried)
1¾ ounces dried echinacea root
10 eucalyptus leaves, shredded
5 ounces fresh shiitake mushrooms, chopped
vodka

Place all the ingredients, except the vodka, loosely in a large, sterilized preserving jar to about two-thirds full. Fill the jar with vodka. Seal the jar, then store in a cool, dark place, shaking the jar every couple of days for a month.

Strain, discarding the plant material and keeping the liquid. Pour the liquid into a sterilized bottle, seal, label, and date.

Take 1 teaspoon in a little water, up to three times a day, as needed.

SHELF LIFE Up to 2 years in a cool, dark place.

THE MUSCULAR SKELETAL SYSTEM

Muscles and bones make up the system that holds us together, moves us around, and allows us to do so much day to day. However, it is easy to take for granted and when something goes wrong, it can be debilitating. Most people have suffered from back, joint, or muscle pain at some point in their life.

Pain can be caused by structural misalignment, and when this happens, visiting a physical therapist, osteopath, or chiropractor is the best approach to treating the root cause. Herbs can help this process and provide further support; for example, anti-inflammatories for muscular pain and nutritional herbs for osteoporosis.

ACTIONS FOR THE MUSCULAR SKELETAL SYSTEM Relaxant, analgesic, anti-inflammatory, circulatory, antiarthritic, antirheumatic, rubefacient.

CRAMPS

A cramp is a painful spasm of the muscles, usually striking at night. It typically affects the foot or calf muscles, but can affect any muscle in the body. If you suffer from frequent cramps, it is best to get it checked out as there can be an underlying reason affecting the area's oxygen supply to the muscles. Use warming, muscle-relaxing herbs for soothing this condition, alongside circulatory stimulants.

HERBS *Crampbark, Ginger, Rosemary, Juniper, Chile, Hawthorn, Yarrow*

MUSCLE AND JOINT PAINS, STRAINS AND SPRAINS

Tendons and ligaments act like elastic bands to hold things together; tendons attach muscle to bone, and ligaments attach bones to each other. Damage to muscles, tendons, and ligaments is usually caused by sudden physical injury, such as twisting an ankle, or through repetitive use, in cases like tennis elbow. Both can be extremely painful, even debilitating.

Use herbs to heal affected tissues along with anti-inflammatories and circulatory stimulants that bring blood to the area. The top herb for tissue damage is comfrey, which stimulates cell growth and repair; St. John's wort helps with pain, and both herbs are anti-inflammatory.

HERBS *Comfrey, St. John's Wort, Elder leaf, Daisy, Chile, Ginger, Juniper, Crampbark*

BACK PAIN

Back pain may be caused by an underlying structural misalignment due to strain or poor posture and is best treated by a physical therapist. Analyze what the cause may be and look to strengthening the area with exercises. Sciatica is a type of trapped nerve pain that travels from the lower back down the leg to the thigh or even the calf.

Internal anti-inflammatories, such as turmeric, St. John's wort, or meadowsweet can be used, or try the soothing pain liniment opposite.

HERBS *St. John's Wort, Turmeric, Skullcap, Juniper, Crampbark, Meadowsweet, Willow, Chile, Mustard, Black Pepper, Rosemary*

HERBAL MUSCLE SOAK

The salt and herbs in this bath salt work together to relax tired muscles, improve circulation, and ease aches and pains.

$^1/_3$ cup salts of your choice, such as Epsom salts, Dead Sea salts, or pink Himalayan salt
2 teaspoons chopped fresh or dried pine needles
2 teaspoons chopped fresh or dried eucalyptus leaf
2 teaspoons fresh or dried lavender flower heads
2 teaspoons dried daisy heads
10 drops of essential oil of your choice, e.g. rosemary, lavender, mint, eucalyptus

Put the salts and herbs into a blender and pulverize them together. This allows the cell walls of the herbs to be broken down so medicinal properties can be extracted into the bath water. Transfer the mixture to a glass or ceramic bowl, add the essential oil and mix well.

To use, add the mixture to a square of cheesecloth. Tie into a bundle at the top with string and then tie this to your hot water bath tap, allowing it to sit just below the tap. Run the hot water directly over and through the bundle, allowing the salt to dissolve and the herbs to be retained inside the cheesecloth (so preventing drain blockage).

Add cold water to the bath to the desired temperature. Soak and relax in the bath for at least 30 minutes.

TIP This mix can be made in bulk (with dried herbs) and stored in a sealed jar in a cool, dark place for up to 1 year.

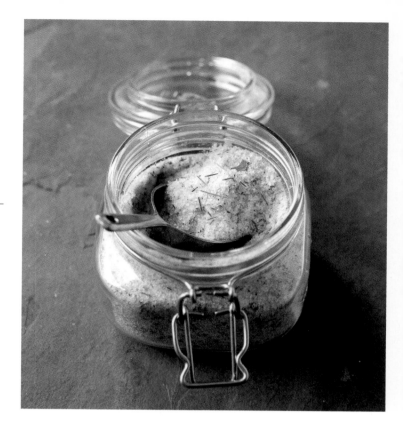

MUSCLE PAIN LINIMENT

This liniment combines the nerve-soothing and pain-relieving properties of St. John's wort, meadowsweet, and willow bark with warming ginger and juniper, to help ease back and sciatic pains. It is also ideal for aching joints and muscles.

$^1/_2$ cup St. John's wort–infused oil
$^1/_2$ cup meadowsweet- or willow bark–infused oil
$^1/_4$ cup juniper and ginger–infused oil
$^2/_3$ cup crampbark tincture
15 drops of rosemary essential oil

Place all the ingredients in a dark glass bottle and seal, then shake well to mix. Label and date.

To use, shake well to mix thoroughly, then massage into the affected area, as needed.

SHELF LIFE Up to 6 months in a cool, dark place.

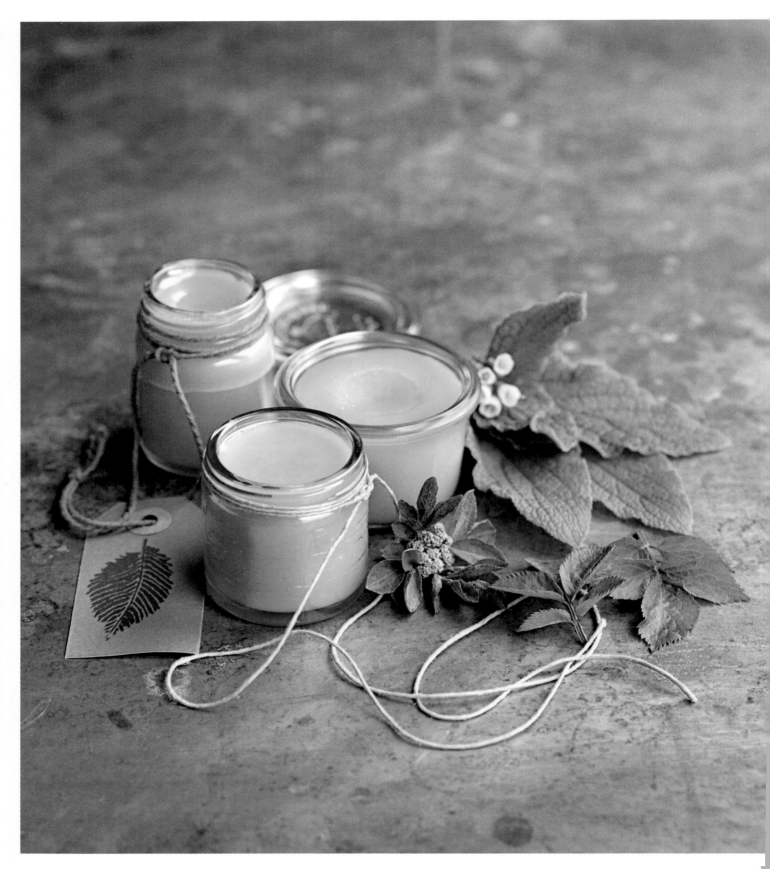

COMFREY AND ELDER BALM

A healing balm for aches, sprains and bruises.

1½ ounces beeswax
⅔ cup comfrey-infused oil
⅔ cup elder leaf-infused oil
20 drops of wintergreen essential oil
10 drops of marjoram essential oil
10 drops of lavender essential oil

Melt the beeswax in a bain-marie, then add the infused oils and mix well until fully combined. Remove from the heat and leave to cool for 5 minutes, then add the essential oils and stir well. Pour into jars, seal, label, and date.

To use, massage into the affected area up to three times a day for a maximum of 2 months at a time.

SHELF LIFE Up to 1 year in a cool, dark place.

BROKEN BONES

Poultices, compresses, or ointments of comfrey and elder can be used to shorten healing time and increase the strength in the fracture site. Traditionally, comfrey leaf and horsetail infusions or tinctures were given internally for a maximum of six weeks, but there are current concerns over certain chemicals found in comfrey, so advice should be sought with an herbalist first. External preparations are more suitable for home use; try the Comfrey and Elder Balm above.

HERBS *Comfrey, Horsetail, Oats, Elder leaf*

ARTHRITIS AND RHEUMATISM

There are two main types of arthritis—osteo and rheumatoid. Both are inflammatory and can be painful and debilitating, requiring different approaches to treat the underlying cause. Osteoarthritis is caused by the general wear and tear of joints that can result in painful inflammation. Rheumatoid arthritis is an autoimmune condition where the joints are attacked by inflammatory

chemicals in an overreactive immune system.

With arthritic conditions, it is important to remove any foods that may be causing inflammation, such as sugar, wheat, dairy, alcohol, and caffeine, while increasing fresh fruits and vegetables and drinking plenty of water.

Foods high in oxalic acid should be researched and avoided; these include spinach and rhubarb. Herbs high in the cooling, anti-inflammatory, and pain-relieving salicylic acids are indicated here—white willow bark and meadowsweet are the herbs of choice. Use them internally, or make a strong bath to bathe inflamed joints. Use herbs that cleanse the body of toxins, particularly herbs that help stimulate the lymphatic system and liver, such as docks, dandelion and cleavers. If pain is preventing sleep, take a nighttime sleep mix that includes calming herbs such as vervain, Californian poppy or wild lettuce.

INTERNAL HERBS *Meadowsweet, Willow bark, Turmeric, Cleavers, Nettle, Yarrow, Vervain, Rosehip, Ginger, Curly Dock, Burdock, Dandelion*

EXTERNAL HERBS *Comfrey, Elder leaf, Ginger, Chile, Black Pepper, Mustard*

OSTEOPOROSIS

Osteoporosis is a weakening in bone density and is generally found in women after menopausal age due to the change in hormones, particularly estrogen, which helps the body retain calcium (see the Female Reproductive System on pages 50–53). It can also be caused by a lack of vitamin D, inadequate absorption of calcium, or certain medications. It can cause an increased risk of osteoarthritis, breaks, and fractures, so needs to be carefully assessed and the underlying causes discovered. Mineral-rich vegetables and herbs should be included in the diet, particularly dandelion leaves, chicory, spinach, and watercress. Bone broth helps to supply the body with bioavailable bone and cartilage strengthening minerals to help maintain bone health (see Chicken Bone Broth on page 56).

HERBS *Horsetail, Nettle, Oats, Red Clover, Dandelion*

THE NERVOUS SYSTEM

The nervous system is the communications center of the body. Consisting of the brain, spinal cord, nerves, and sensory organs, it connects all the other body systems, processing huge amounts of information at lightning speed.

Stress can have a huge impact on our nervous system and overall health. A certain amount of stress helps us function when we are under pressure, keeps us alert and focused, motivates us to achieve, and keeps us safe when danger looms. But when stress is extreme or long-term it can have damaging effects on our health. This is because the nervous system can have difficulty distinguishing between life-threatening stress and everyday stresses, meaning that our bodies can remain in a constant fight or flight mode.

Long exposure to the stress hormones cortisol, adrenaline, and noradrenaline can cause an imbalance of hormones in the blood. This in turn disrupts blood sugar levels and immune cells, making the body more susceptible to a whole host of illnesses including diabetes, high blood pressure, poor concentration, memory problems, headaches, sleep disturbance, and anxiety.

To lessen the effects of chronic external stress, we must keep our nervous system in peak condition. Our brain and nerves require a constant supply of high-quality proteins and fats, particularly the essential fatty acid omega-3, as well as B vitamins, magnesium, and potassium. All these nutrients help to keep our neurons firing.

While external stressors are usually out of our control, we can have a direct, conscious influence over the nervous system, putting ourselves in control of our body's response to stress. Find what de-stresses you—breathing exercises, yoga, or walks in the woods (perhaps gather some herbs)—and do it often to reset your stress levels. Regular exercise lifts the mood and supplies the brain with adequate oxygen to function and perform; when our brains and bodies function at a high level, we can cope better with daily tasks and stressors.

Adaptogenic herbs do what their name suggests; they help the body to adapt to stress, supporting the nervous system and adrenals—the glands mainly responsible for stress hormones. Try licorice and skullcap tea to restore vitality.

Nervines and anxiolytics; for example, skullcap, oat straw, rose, and vervain, help the body to relax and rejuvenate. They calm the mind and help reduce the physical effects of stress such as palpitations, insomnia, and headaches.

ACTIONS FOR THE NERVOUS SYSTEM Nervine, anxiolytic, adaptogen, sedative, stimulant, tonic, antispasmodic, antidepressant, analgesic, liver cleansing.

ANXIETY

A feeling of worry or unease is something everyone experiences at some point in life. When extreme, anxiety can even cause the physical symptoms of palpitations, rapid breathing, sweating, and tension. Self-care and relaxation techniques are invaluable here. Take some time to brew a cup of herbal tea, sit quietly, sip, and breathe deeply. Try the "connecting with the breath" exercise on page 76.

HERBS *Motherwort, Skullcap, Lemon Balm, Oat straw, Chamomile, Linden blossom, Vervain, Hawthorn, Poppy, Rose, Lavender, Rosemary*

DEPRESSION AND LOW MOOD

Depression and low mood can be caused or exacerbated by external factors or by internal thought processes. While the underlying cause must be addressed, herbs can help to lift the mood in mild to moderate depression.

HERBS *St. John's Wort, Skullcap, Linden blossom, Nettle seed, Rose, Vervain*

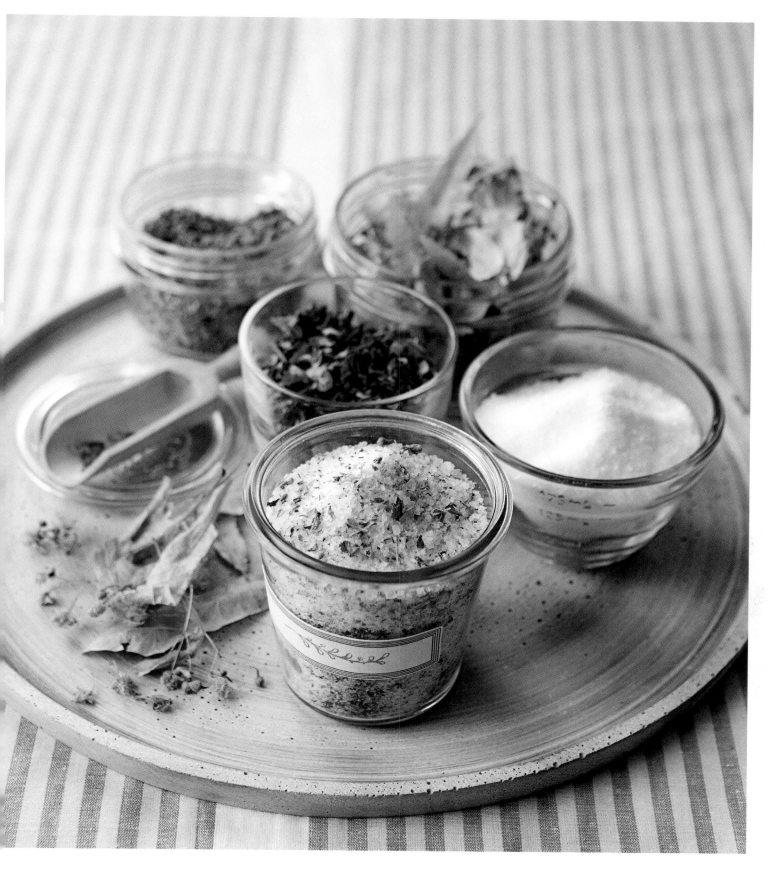

RELAXING HERBAL BATH RECIPE

This recipe uses a strong infusion of anxiety-reducing herbs. The Epsom salts combat physical tension by relaxing the muscles. If you cannot find Epsom salts, replace with Dead Sea salts.

3½ ounces Epsom salts
¾ ounce fresh or dried linden blossom
5 drops of lavender essential oil
5 drops of rose essential oil

Put the salts and linden blossom into a blender and pulverize them together. This allows the cell walls of the herb to be broken down so the scents and medicinal properties can be extracted in the bath water. Transfer the mixture to a glass or ceramic bowl, add the essential oils, and mix well.

To use, add the mixture to a square of cheesecloth. Tie into a bundle at the top with string and then tie this to your hot water bath tap, allowing it to sit just below the tap. Run the hot water directly over and through the bundle, allowing the salts to dissolve and the herbs to be retained inside the cheesecloth (so preventing drain blockage).

Add cold water to the bath to the desired temperature. Soak and relax in the bath for at least 30 minutes.

TIP This mix can be made in bulk (with dried herbs) and stored in a sealed jar in a cool, dark place for up to 1 year.

MOOD LIFT TEA

With depression, it is important to take time for self-care. Take a moment to make a healing, herbal tea at least once a day to help lift the spirits.

1¾ ounces dried rose
1¾ ounces dried skullcap
1¾ ounces dried St. John's wort
1¾ ounces dried vervain

Pour all the herbs into a sterilized jar and shake to mix them together. Seal, label, and date.

Make an infusion with 1–2 teaspoons of the dried herb in 1 cup of boiling water, cover, and steep for 15 minutes. Strain and drink.

Drink up to three times per day.

SHELF LIFE Keep the dried herb mix in a cool, dark place for up to 1 year.

CAUTION Check with an herbalist before taking St John's wort with other medications.

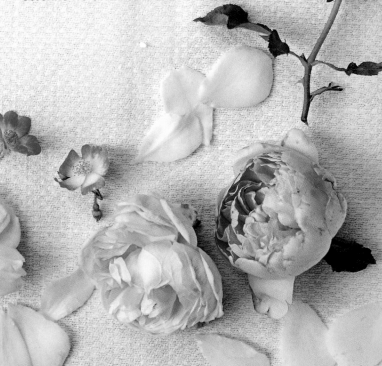

HEADACHES

Many things can cause headaches: stress, muscle tension, eyestrain, circulatory dysfunction, digestive disorders, hormonal factors . . . the list goes on. Finding the underlying cause where headaches are chronic and frequent may be a job for a health-care professional, but herbs can certainly help to soothe and lessen the pain. A few drops of lavender and peppermint essential oil in a steam inhalation, or diluted in base oil and rubbed on the temples and forehead, can cool and soothe a headache.

Herbs that relax the nervous system, improve circulation, and reduce pain can lessen headache attacks and severity. Wood betony and feverfew are specific herbs for headaches. Combine them with other appropriate herbs for your symptoms; for example, relaxants such as crampbark if there is muscle tension, or red clover for hormone balancing.

HERBS *Wood Betony, Feverfew, Meadowsweet, Willow bark, Yarrow, Chamomile, Linden blossom, Poppy, Crampbark, Lavender, Peppermint, Basil*

INSOMNIA

Insomnia is commonly associated with stress, anxiety, tension, and an inability to shut down after the day's stimulation. Try to have a wind-down period before bed, without electronic screens. Take time for relaxing herbal baths, self-massage, and mindfulness. Lack of sleep can directly impact on the body's ability to regenerate and heal and is a contributing factor to many diseases. Nervine herbs encourage the body and mind to relax, aiding a peaceful sleep. Sedative herbs like Californian poppy and wild lettuce both induce sleep; these can be used for acute insomnia due to travel, for example, or for short periods of stress. Try the Chamomile Bedtime Latte on page 127 or the Golden Milk recipe to the right.

HERBS *Linden blossom, Chamomile, Skullcap, Poppy, Wild Lettuce, St. John's Wort, Lavender*

LOW ENERGY

A feeling of constant low energy is a sign that something is out of balance; the body is not working at its full capacity and so you can feel drained, both physically and emotionally. The familiar plant-based stimulants coffee and tea have a marked effect on energy levels and are helpful for increasing energy in very short-term situations—pulling an all-nighter to meet a study or work deadline is something many of us are guilty of. Adaptogenic herbs can be used long-term in place of these stimulants, to nourish the nervous system and improve energy levels.

HERBS *Nettle seed, Skullcap, Licorice, Rosemary, Holy Basil. See also Adaptogens for the Nervous System box on page 67.*

GOLDEN MILK

This golden tonic milk is based on a traditional Ayurvedic recipe. Made with anti-inflammatory turmeric and sedative poppy seeds (these nourish the nervous system, aiding in a peaceful night's sleep), along with cardamom and vanilla, it soothes and relaxes the muscles and mind. Drink a mugful before bed to slip into a deep slumber.

1 mugful (about 1 cup) almond or oat milk
1 teaspoon freshly grated turmeric or turmeric powder
1 teaspoon ground poppy seeds
½ cinnamon stick
3 cardamom pods
½ vanilla pod (or ½ teaspoon vanilla extract)
1 teaspoon coconut oil
1–2 teaspoons honey or unrefined sugar (optional)

Combine the milk, turmeric, poppy seeds, cinnamon, cardamom, and vanilla in a saucepan, bring to a simmer, cover, and turn the heat off. Leave to steep for 5–10 minutes, strain the mixture into a mug, and then stir in the coconut oil and honey or sugar (if using). Serve, stirring between sips.

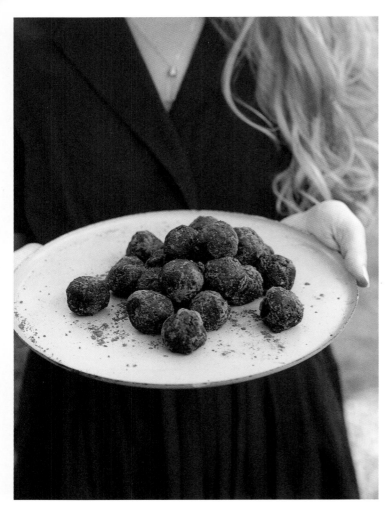

NEURALGIA

Neuralgia is pain that follows the path of a nerve, commonly affecting the lower back, head, or neck. The underlying cause is damage or inflammation to the nerve fibers usually through injury or viral infection such as shingles. Pain levels can range from excruciatingly constant to intermittent twinges.

The current orthodox treatment of neuralgia focuses around painkillers, which may be necessary when pain is debilitating or chronic. A diet high in B vitamins and omega-3 fatty acids can provide the building blocks the body needs to repair the damage.

Herbal treatment uses anti-inflammatory analgesic, nervine, and vulnerary herbs to help the repair process. If sleep is affected by pain, a soothing nervine tea before bed may help (see the Insomnia section on page 65). Massaging the area with St. John's wort oil or Comfrey and Elder Balm (see page 61) helps loosen tight muscles, lessen pain and inflammation, and heal tissue.

EXTERNAL HERBS *St. John's Wort, Comfrey, Elder leaf, Chile, Ginger, Juniper, Rosemary, Lavender*
INTERNAL HERBS *Linden blossom, St John's Wort, Skullcap, Oat straw, Poppy*

ENERGY BALLS

These energy balls combine nutritive almonds, cocoa, coconut, and pumpkin seeds with adaptogenic nettle seed to tone the nervous system and restore natural vitality.

¾ ounce fresh nettle seed
a handful of fresh or dried nettle leaf
6 ounces pitted dates
2½ ounces blanched almonds
1¾ ounces pumpkin seeds
1½ tablespoons coconut oil
¼ cup cocoa powder
desiccated coconut or cocoa powder, for coating

Blend all the ingredients, except the desiccated coconut, together in a food processor. Alternatively, grind them in batches using a mortar and pestle, then combine.

Roll the resulting paste into balls, each about ¾ inch in diameter, and coat with desiccated coconut or cocoa powder. Store in an airtight container in the fridge.

Eat 1–2 balls a day.

SHELF LIFE These will keep in the fridge for up to 2 weeks, or they can be frozen for up to 6 months (defrost before serving).

SHINGLES

Shingles is an infection caused by a latent chickenpox virus reemerging in a nerve of the body. It usually appears on one side only, and often affects the torso or neck. Little blisters appear on the skin; these are infectious and can be incredibly painful.

Treat shingles internally with immune-boosting and antiviral herbs such as echinacea, elderberry, and St. John's wort. Because the lesions can be extremely painful, soak cotton swabs with infusions or diluted tinctures and dab the area rather than rub. Alternatively, use a spray bottle. When blisters begin to heal, use St. John's wort–infused oil to gently massage the affected areas and reduce nerve damage.

INTERNAL HERBS *St. John's Wort, Echinacea, Elderberry, Thyme, Eucalyptus*
EXTERNAL HERBS *St. John's Wort, Chickweed, Lavender, Thyme, Lemon Balm*

ADAPTOGENS FOR THE NERVOUS SYSTEM

Nervous system adaptogens allow the body to "adapt" to environmental stress, both emotional and physical. They increase overall vitality, and aid the body's general capacity to withstand stress and the diseases associated with it. Many herbs here may not be found in the wild but are important for working with stress. Find them in health food stores or through an herbalist.

CENTELLA ASIATICA–GOTU KOLA, BRAHMI

ACTIONS Adaptogen, anxiolytic, wound healing, alterative.
INDICATIONS Poor memory, skin and tissue damage, acne, scarring, connective tissue diseases, cellulite.
Gotu kola is excellent for healing all connective tissues; it can be used for arthritis and joint problems and wound healing. It is used in Ayurveda and Chinese medicine traditions for longevity and improving memory.

PANAX GINSENG–KOREAN GINSENG

ACTIONS Adaptogen, cardioprotective, liver tonic, anti-inflammatory, immune modulator, tonic.
INDICATIONS Weakness and debility, convalescence, poor concentration, low mood, immune deficiency, cardiovascular disease.
Panax ginseng helps to improve physical and mental performance and is often used by athletes to improve stamina and recovery time. It also has blood pressure lowering effects.

SCHISANDRA CHINENSIS–SCHISANDRA, FIVE-FLAVOR BERRY

ACTIONS Adaptogen, bitter, liver tonic, nerve tonic, antioxidant.
INDICATIONS Insomnia, chronic fatigue, poor memory, low mood, liver clearance.
Schisandra is an energizing adaptogen, increasing energy levels without being overly stimulating. It improves concentration and memory, especially for those who have scattered thoughts.

WITHANIA SOMNIFERA–ASHWAGANDHA, INDIAN GINSENG, WINTER CHERRY

ACTIONS Adaptogen, sedative, tonic, nervine, heart tonic, hypotensive, nourishing.
INDICATIONS Convalescence, weakness and debility, nervous exhaustion, low libido.
Withania is a building, nourishing, and restorative adaptogen. It benefits those who have lost weight due to illness and will strengthen a weak constitution. It is not used for acute infections.
OTHER NERVOUS SYSTEM ADAPTOGENS Rosemary, nettle, skullcap (see their individual sections).

THE SKIN

Our skin is an amazing organ and is so much more than just a covering. It is a semiporous, infection-fighting, self-healing ecosystem, filled with nerve endings that allow us to interact with our outside world. It keeps the things we need in and the things we don't out.

The skin is the largest and most visible organ of the body. From a holistic viewpoint, it is a useful indicator of our internal health. It works with our other eliminatory organs—the kidneys, liver, bowels, and lungs—to maintain homeostasis, regulating body temperature and hydration levels and excreting metabolic wastes.

When healthy, the body is in a constant state of detoxification and, contrary to health fashion, it usually does not require special "detox" diets or supplements. However, when there is an extra burden on the eliminatory organs from an illness or allergy, for example, it may be necessary to give the body a gentle nudge to restore balance. In herbal medicine, the first port of call for almost any skin condition is to use bitter herbs and alteratives. Bitters stimulate the liver and digestion, helping to clear toxins from the body, while alteratives aid the lymphatic system to clear away infection and wastes.

The well-known sayings "you are what you eat" and "beauty starts within" are particularly true when we consider the skin. When the body is in a state of health and vitality, our skin glows. Eating a varied, whole food diet low in refined sugars and fried foods does wonders for the complexion. For example, anti-inflammatory flavonoids found in colorful fruits and vegetables bring down redness and help repair free radical damage. Drinking lots of water and herb teas keeps us hydrated and helps maintain the integrity of the skin, so up your veggies, up your water intake and you'll soon notice the difference.

Long-term, chronic skin conditions can be hard to shift. To truly get to the bottom of a skin disorder we must think holistically and consider a number of possible contributing factors. We must assess internal health, external triggers, such as allergens and irritants, as well as the emotional state of a person. If your eczema is caused by an allergen to wheat or dairy, cut them out of your diet. If your hives are caused by anxiety, practice relaxation techniques and take nervines and soothing herbs. Treat the cause of the disease.

ACTIONS FOR THE SKIN Alterative, lymphatic stimulant, liver clearance, wound and tissue healer, antimicrobial.

ACNE

Most commonly affecting the face, chest, and back, acne is caused by an overproduction of sebum, which blocks hair follicles, causing spots to develop on the skin. One of the main causes of excess sebum is hormonal imbalance, particularly where there is a surge of testosterone as seen in adolescents and polycystic ovarian syndrome (PCOS). It is therefore important to address any underlying hormonal issues (see also Herbs for the Female Reproductive System on page 50).

Diet and gut health are also an important factor as a sluggish system may result in the reuptake of waste hormones and toxins. Support the liver and digestion with bitter herbs such as dandelion and burdock root to help clear toxins in the blood. Lymphatic herbs encourage the removal of wastes and infection, while topical antimicrobials and vulneraries bring down redness and reduce scaring.

INTERNAL HERBS *Burdock, Calendula, Cleavers, Chickweed, Dandelion, Echinacea, Nettle, Willow bark, Curly Dock, Licorice, Chamomile*
EXTERNAL HERBS *Aloe Vera, Berberis, Witch Hazel, Lavender, Calendula, Yarrow, Comfrey, Meadowsweet, Chamomile*

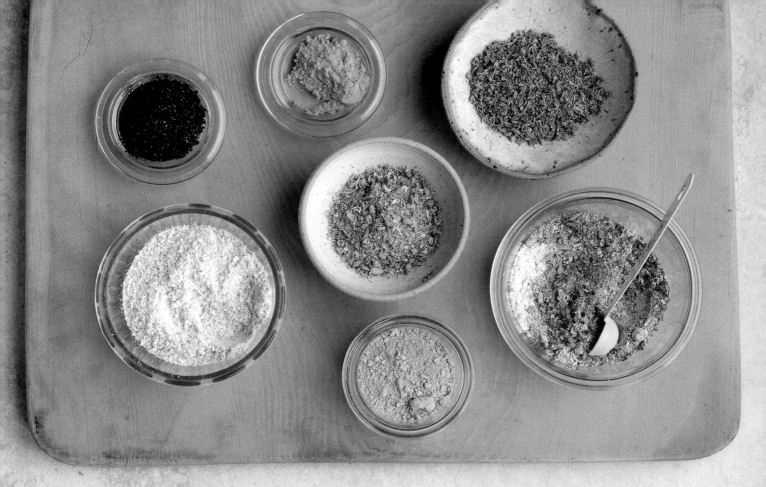

GENTLE 3 IN 1 CLEANSER

Overly harsh facial washes and wipes can dry out the skin, causing it to overproduce sebum. This multitasking face wash acts as a cleanser, exfoliant, and mask. Anti-inflammatory yarrow, chamomile and turmeric calm irritated skin, while green clay draws out excess dirt and sebum. The dried herbs and ground berries gently exfoliate to prevent blocked pores.

1 tablespoon finely ground oats or almonds

1 tablespoon green clay (other clays such as red, kaolin, or rhassoul work well too)

1 tablespoon finely ground dried herbs—a mix of chamomile and yarrow flowers

2 teaspoons finely ground dried berberis berries or elderberries

1 teaspoon turmeric powder

Combine all the ingredients in a jar. Seal. Shake. Label. Date. Voilà!

Place a heaping teaspoon in your palm, add a few drops of water, and mix into a paste. If you have dry or sensitive skin, add a few drops of glycerin or honey to the mix.

Rub all over your face and neck in a circular motion, leave on for 5 minutes, and then wash off.

SHELF LIFE Keep in a cool, dry place for up to 1 year or more (provided it's kept in a dry environment).

WILLOW SKIN CALMING SERUM

White willow contains anti-inflammatory compounds that reduce redness and bring down infection. Chamomile and yarrow essential oils are also potent anti-inflammatory agents, while lemon is clarifying and toning.

3 tablespoons organic aloe vera gel
1–2 teaspoons cold-pressed grapeseed or jojoba oil
5 drops of pure vitamin E oil
1 teaspoon white willow bark tincture
5 drops of chamomile blue or yarrow essential oil
5 drops of lemon essential oil
5 drops of frankincense essential oil

Note: Usually fresh is best, but for this recipe the aloe must be bought premixed as it needs an emulsifier to blend with the other ingredients.

Place the aloe vera gel in a bowl, then slowly add the grapeseed and vitamin E oils, drop by drop, whisking constantly to emulsify the mixture; the more oil you add, the more moisturizing the serum will be, but it can be left out altogether, if you prefer.

Once the oil is well mixed in, slowly add the willow tincture, whisking well. Finally, mix in the essential oils.

Transfer to a sterilized bottle (a pump bottle is the best option for this serum), then seal, label, and date.

Use as a light, astringent moisturizer, or with a cotton ball as a lotion-type cleanser.

SHELF LIFE Keep in a cool, dry place for up to 6 months.

DRAWING OINTMENT

Drawing ointments help to "draw" out infection and pus from spots and splinters, bringing them to a head. If you don't see improvement after a week, seek professional medical advice.

¾ ounce marshmallow root powder or slippery elm powder
¾ ounce bentonite clay
¾ teaspoon honey
2 to 4 tablespoons herbal infusion (choose from list of external herbs in Abscesses and Boils opposite)

Blend all the ingredients together in a bowl to form a paste, adding just enough of the herbal infusion to get a good, thick paste-like consistency.

To use, apply the paste thickly to the affected area; cover with a Band-Aid or bandage. Leave in place for up to 6 hours before refreshing and changing the ointment as necessary.

SHELF LIFE Store in an airtight container in the fridge and use within 3 days.

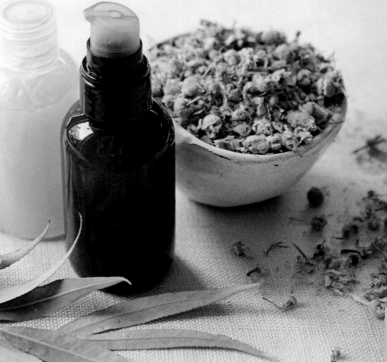

ABSCESSES AND BOILS

These are both a localized skin infection usually caused by bacteria, which create a buildup of pus under the skin. Simple boils should clear up on their own in a couple of weeks but can be helped along with home care. Alterative and anti-infective herbs can be used internally to help clear infection. Antibacterial and wound-healing herbs can be used externally, especially in the form of drawing ointments and poultices, as they can help bring the boil to a head.

INTERNAL HERBS *Echinacea, Burdock, Berberis, Calendula, Cleavers, Curly Dock*

EXTERNAL HERBS *Plantain, Calendula, Marshmallow, Comfrey leaf poultice, Lavender, Thyme*

BITES AND STINGS

To bring down itching and irritation from insect bites, apply fresh, mucilaginous herbs such as aloe or chickweed to soothe the area. Anti-inflammatory herbs can be used for stings; a compress of fresh crushed calendula or plantain works well. If you don't have fresh herbs on hand, apply some of the Soothing Skin Cream (see page 72).

EXTERNAL HERBS *Calendula, Aloe Vera, Plantain, Chickweed, Lavender*

BRUISES

Bruises are bluish purple marks caused by broken blood vessels under the skin, usually from an impact, which should resolve itself in a week or two. Arnica is a popular remedy for bruising and can be bought over the counter in ointment form, but Comfrey and Elder Balm (see page 61) is just as effective and more likely to be found in a hedge near you! Alternatively, a poultice of any of the herbs below will help strengthen the blood vessels and heal bruising.

CAUTION If bruises are very large or frequent, seek medical attention.

EXTERNAL HERBS *Elder leaf, Comfrey, Yarrow, Witch Hazel*

BURNS

For minor sunburn and heat burns, aloe vera is a great herb to have on hand, especially when used fresh from the plant; simply smear all over the affected area. A few drops of calendula-infused oil and lavender essential oil also add a moisturizing and antiseptic effect.

EXTERNAL HERBS *Calendula, Aloe, Witch Hazel, Lavender, Chickweed*

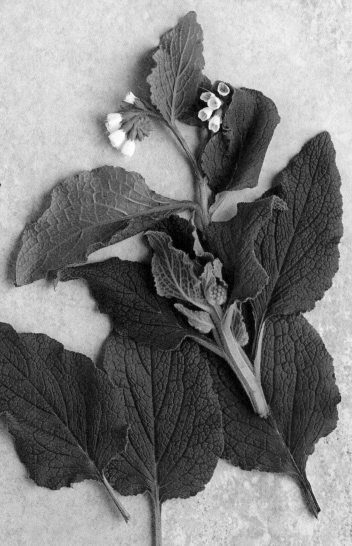

CHILBLAINS

Chilblains are swelling, redness, and pain on the fingers and toes caused by inflammation of the blood vessels when exposed to the cold. See the Cardiovascular System on page 36.

ECZEMA

Eczema and dermatitis are both terms used to describe inflammatory skin conditions causing itchy patches anywhere on the body. Eczema is most commonly found around the knees, elbows, neck, and hands and is usually caused by an allergy; identifying and avoiding the allergen can help alleviate the condition. People with allergic skin conditions may find that it worsens around periods of stress, in which case drinking soothing, nervine herbal teas may be helpful. Take alterative, bitter, and lymphatic herbs internally to aid the body's elimination of wastes that may exacerbate this inflammatory skin condition.

Topically, moisturizing creams can soothe irritation and prevent damage to the skin from scratching; try the Soothing Skin Cream recipe, right. Cutting out harsh soaps and synthetic skin products can also help reduce irritation; try using mucilaginous oats to soften hard water to wash with. Simply tie the oats up in some cheesecloth or an old stocking, run under hot water, and use as you would a sponge.

INTERNAL HERBS *Dandelion root, Burdock root, Cleavers, Berberis, Calendula, Nettle, Licorice, Skullcap*
EXTERNAL HERBS *Calendula, Chickweed, Comfrey, Rosehip oil, Plantain, Oats, Aloe, Licorice*

SOOTHING SKIN CREAM

This cream can be used for inflamed skin conditions of all kinds, and it is especially useful for eczema, burns, rashes, and wounds to reduce scarring.

¾ ounce emulsifying wax
⅓ ounce beeswax
3 tablespoons chickweed-infused oil
½ cup chamomile infusion
¼ cup aloe vera gel
¼ cup calendula tincture
20 drops of lavender essential oil
½ teaspoon pure vitamin E oil
preservative of your choice (optional)

Melt the waxes and chickweed-infused oil together in a bain-marie. Gently heat the chamomile infusion, aloe gel, and calendula tincture together in a separate saucepan.

Remove both mixtures from the heat. You want to try to get the two mixtures to around the same temperature before combining them. The easiest way to do this is to heat them, then leave them to cool to around blood temperature (98.6°F) before combining—the oils will cool more slowly than the infusion, so you may need to gently reheat the infusion again before combining the two. (Alternatively, you can use a cooking thermometer to measure the temperature of both mixtures during heating, until they reach the same temperature.)

Pour the chamomile mix slowly, bit by bit, into the combined wax and oil, whisking constantly with a handheld electric mixer. Keep whisking until the cream begins to cool and thicken. Mix in the essential oil, vitamin E, and preservative (if using).

Place in a sterilized jar, seal, label, and date.

To use, apply to affected areas, as needed.

SHELF LIFE This cream will last up to 3 months if kept in the fridge; adding a preservative will extend the shelf life up to 1 year.

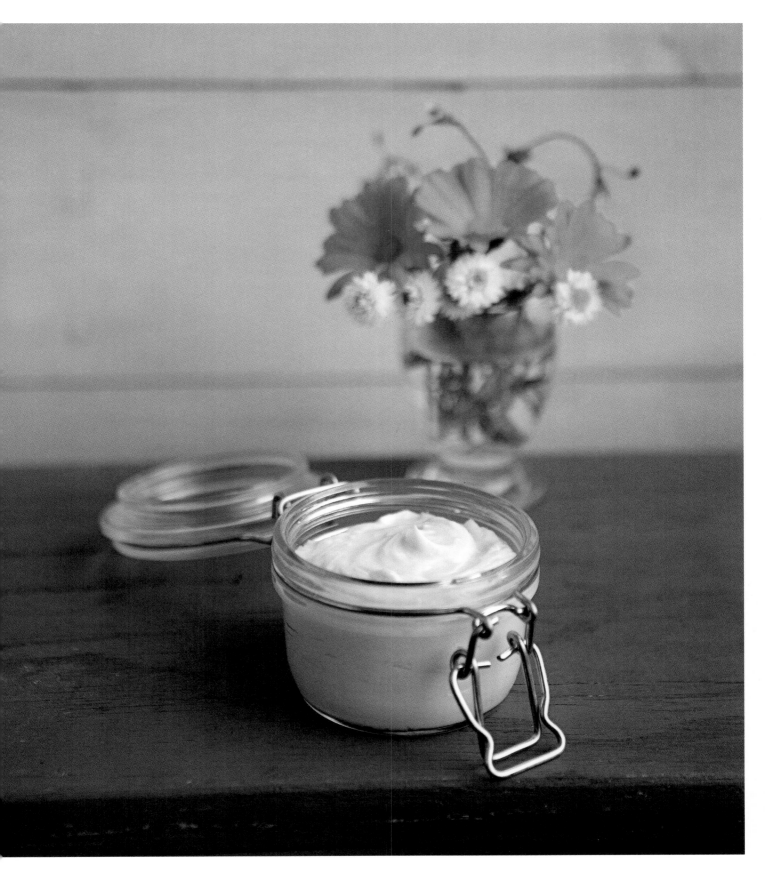

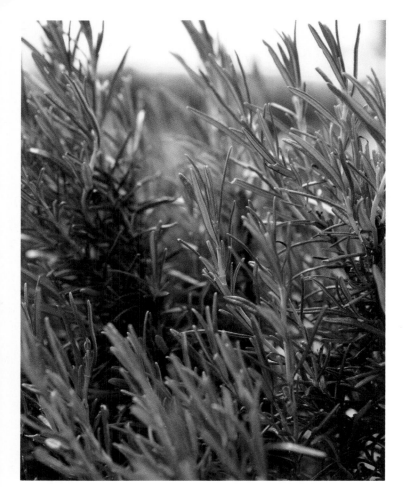

HAIR TONIC

This hair rinse contains mineral-rich herbs including rosemary, sage, and nettle. It is antifungal and stimulates circulation in the scalp, helping to clear away flakiness and give a lustrous shine to the hair. Ideal for dandruff, psoriasis of the scalp, and for dull, brittle hair.

a handful of fresh or dried nettle leaves
a handful of fresh or dried rosemary leaves
a handful of fresh or dried sage leaves
1 quart boiling water
¼ cup organic apple cider vinegar

Put the herbs into a bowl, pour over the boiling water, and leave to infuse and cool to a comfortable temperature, then strain out the herbs. Add the cider vinegar to the remaining liquid.

To use, after washing and rinsing hair, pour all of the hair tonic over your hair as a final rinse; there is no need to wash it out. Style hair as usual.

DANDRUFF

Dandruff is characterized by flaky, dry skin on the scalp caused by a number of conditions including fungal infection, allergies, seborrheic dermatitis, psoriasis, eczema, and irritation from harsh shampoos and hair products. It may be tempting to use an anti-dandruff shampoo to wash away the flakiness, but this may cause further irritation. Instead, use a gentle, natural shampoo and follow up with a final rinse of strong herbal tea made with rosemary, sage, and nettle (see Hair Tonic recipe, right).

INTERNAL HERBS *Burdock, Curly Dock, Cleavers, Calendula, Nettle, Dandelion*
EXTERNAL HERBS *Rosemary, Sage, Nettle, Calendula, Eucalyptus, Tea Tree essential oil, Calendula-infused oil*

Rosemary *Rosmarinus officinalis* (above).

FUNGAL INFECTIONS

We have fungi and bacteria all over our bodies, but certain fungi, such as candida, can overgrow, resulting in itching, swelling, and discomfort. Common fungal infections, including ringworm, athlete's foot, and jock's itch, are caused by the Tinea fungi and are spread through close contact. Scrupulous hygiene and antifungal herbs can help prevent spreading and clear up infection. Fungal infections can be quite persistent so long-term treatment may be necessary.

Treat the problem both externally with antifungal herbs, as well as internally with immune-boosting herbs such as echinacea. It is important to let the infected skin breathe and keep it cool, as heat and moisture are prime breeding spots for fungi.

Fungal nails can take years to clear up and may require a more vigorous herbal protocol. Neat tea tree oil, eucalyptus oil, and myrrh tincture can be applied twice daily after soaking the feet in an antifungal herbal foot bath (see Make for herbal bath instructions on page 21).

INTERNAL HERBS *Echinacea, Elderberry, Cleavers, Curly Dock, Thyme, Oregano, Berberis, Calendula*
EXTERNAL HERBS *Calendula, Eucalyptus, Myrrh, Thyme, Oregano, Tea Tree essential oil*

PSORIASIS

Psoriasis is an abnormal production of skin cells resulting in raised patches of dry, inflamed skin. Primarily it is an autoimmune condition with a hereditary link. Stress and emotional health can play a big factor in psoriasis, but identifying the exact trigger can be difficult. To fully treat an autoimmune condition, it may be necessary to seek professional help.

At home remedies that may help include soothing herbs such as those mentioned under Eczema (see page 72), herbs for the nervous system to help with stress, and liver-clearing and alterative herbs. Psoriasis often affects the scalp, in which case, try the Hair Tonic, opposite.

INTERNAL HERBS *Burdock, Cleavers, Dandelion, Curly Dock, Berberis, Red Clover, Calendula, Nettle*
EXTERNAL HERBS *Chickweed, Marshmallow, Cleavers*

ANTIFUNGAL FOOT POWDER

This powder contains powerful antifungal agents that help absorb and prevent excess moisture.

⅓ cup cornstarch
½ cup kaolin or bentonite clay
1 tablespoon finely ground myrrh powder
20 drops of eucalyptus essential oil
20 drops of thyme essential oil

Combine all the ingredients in a container (an old baby powder bottle is perfect if you have one) and cover/seal. Shake well. Label and date.

Use as needed as you would talcum powder.

SHELF LIFE Use within 6 months. Top up with a few more drops of essential oils if the smell fades.

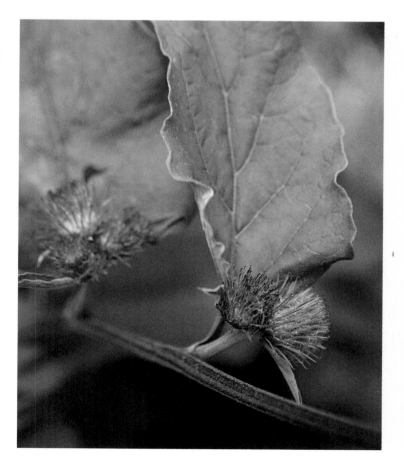

Burdock *Arctium lappa* (right)

THE RESPIRATORY SYSTEM

The basic function of the respiratory system is to exchange gases, swapping waste carbon dioxide with oxygen. Together with the circulatory system, this vital oxygen is delivered to all cells in the body via the blood. Our tissues require a constant supply of oxygen to function properly. Impairment to the airways or the delicate mucous membranes that line them will leave us more prone to disease and disorder. Oxygen is also needed in the reaction to release energy from the food we eat, so poor respiratory health may also affect our overall energy levels and vitality.

The membranes that line the airways produce mucus to filter air, trapping unwanted particles such as bacteria and dust. Herbal treatments of the respiratory system focus on keeping these mucous membranes healthy. When they are dry and irritated, use mucilaginous, demulcent herbs to coat, cool, and soothe the tissues. Conversely, when there is too much mucus, use herbs to gently tone, break up, and remove excess catarrh, such as astringents and expectorants.

The respiratory system is prone to picking up bacteria and viruses such as colds, flu, and chest infections, so treatments should include herbs that boost the immune system and are antimicrobial, like garlic, echinacea, and elderberry.

ACTIONS FOR THE RESPIRATORY SYSTEM Expectorant, antitussive, demulcent, anti-inflammatory, antiviral, antibacterial, immune stimulant.

CONNECTING WITH THE BREATH

"The way that we breathe is the way that we feel" is a wise Ayurvedic saying—breathing fully, deeply, and freely affects our mood and physical health. Take a minute. Think about how you are breathing now. How do your ribs and tummy rise and fall? How far does your breath go into your chest and abdomen? Which muscles are you using?

We are so often in a rush or existing in a state of stress that our breath can become rapid and shallow. If you feel you suffer from poor breathing patterns, try some deep breathing exercises. Any form of exercise will increase your breathing ability and enhance your oxygen supply. At the very least, stop once a day and take a few minutes to concentrate on deep breathing. You may find your energy levels rise and your stress levels decrease.

COUGHS AND CHEST INFECTIONS

Coughing is a natural reflex to get rid of mucus and substances that should not be in the airways. Some coughs are dry and nonproductive; these are usually caused by allergies or irritation. Some are "wet" and phlegmy and are usually the result of infection. Treat the infection and boost the immune system with herbs such as garlic, echinacea, and elderberry.

Addressing any underlying allergies or irritants can help dry coughs. Mucilaginous and antitussive herbs help to soothe irritation and inflammation and relax the airways. This is particularly useful when a dry cough is preventing a restful and healing night's sleep.

Where there is a cough with a lot of mucus, herbs can be used to encourage the removal of infection and phlegm. Mucolytic herbs thin the mucus, and expectorants gently encourage the cough reflex, easing the strain; examples of these are thyme and elecampane.

Herbs for coughs are ideally taken in soothing syrups that coat and "stick" to the respiratory tract. Make a cough syrup using the basic syrup recipe on page 78. An effective and traditional recipe includes dried licorice root, fresh thyme, and elderberries. Support the immune system internally with herbs such as echinacea and elderberry to battle infection at the same time.

HERBS *Garlic, Elecampane, Wild Cherry bark, Thyme, Licorice, Linden blossom, Marshmallow, Echinacea, Elderberry, Thyme, Sage, Violet, Angelica*

SORE THROATS

Sore throats are usually the signal of the start of a cold or flu, but can develop into more severe infections such as laryngitis or tonsillitis. There are a variety of traditional remedies you can reach for: try gargling with a strong sage decoction or a diluted sage and blackberry leaf–infused vinegar. Fragrant honeysuckle blossoms can be infused in honey, combining antiviral and pain-killing properties. Another excellent remedy is the pain-busting throat spray on page 110, or try the Elderflower, Lemon, and Ginger Cough Drops on page 79.

HERBS *Sage, Blackberry, Honeysuckle, Echinacea, Elderflower, Elderberry*

CONGESTION AND SINUSITIS

Congestion is caused by a mucus buildup in the cavities of the upper airways and can leave you feeling stuffy. Steam inhalations with aromatic, antimicrobial herbs are a great way to get the healing action of herbs direct to the airway and relieve symptoms.

Severe congestion can block the sinus passages and leave you with sinusitis—an inflamed, tender, painful face and eye area. Steam inhalations can also be of use here, and so can astringent herbs; a tea made of plantain and ground ivy can clear stuffiness and ease pain.

Sinus pain usually resolves once the underlying infection has cleared up but can sometimes become a chronic condition. There is evidence to suggest that chronic sinusitis may be associated with a dairy sensitivity or a fungal infection. In this case, remove dairy from the diet and take herbal tinctures or teas that are immune-boosting, such as echinacea or elderberry, along with antifungals, such as thyme and oregano.

HERBS *Ground Ivy, Plantain, Elderflower, Elderberry, Echinacea, Oregano, Eucalyptus, Thyme, Sage, Basil*

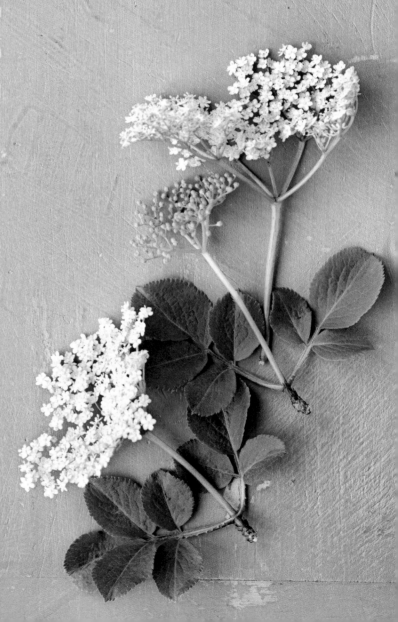

DECONGESTANT CHEST RUB

Elder leaf helps to ease aching muscles from strained breathing and coughing and is antiviral. The aromatic essential oils add a clearing and opening action for helping clear congestion.

a handful of fresh spring elder leaves
¼ cup organic coconut oil
10 drops of thyme essential oil
15 drops of eucalyptus essential oil
15 drops of lavender essential oil

Place the fresh spring elder leaves and coconut oil in a bain-marie. Gently heat for 30 minutes, until the oil is a light green color.

Remove from the heat, straining the leaves out, and leave to cool slightly, then stir in the essential oils.

Pour into a jar and leave to set. Place the lid on, label, and date.

To use, rub over the chest and back area as needed.

SHELF LIFE Up to 1 year in a cool, dark place.

QUICK ONION AND HONEY COUGH SYRUP

Use the antimicrobial action of garlic and onions with the sweet and healing properties of honey to soothe all types of coughs. It is surprisingly tasty!

1 onion
1 garlic clove (optional, but can make it strong tasting!)
honey or unrefined sugar, to cover

Peel and roughly chop the onion and garlic (if using) and place in a sterilized jar. Pour enough honey over the onion to cover it. If using sugar, alternately layer ½ inch onion with enough sugar to cover; repeat until the jar is full or the onion is used up.

Cover and leave for at least 30 minutes, after which time you can use the runny liquid as a syrup. Ideally the mixture will be left at least overnight, but even better, prepare it in advance and leave it to infuse for up to a week (in a cool, dark place) before straining.

Strain the liquid into a clean sterilized jar before use. Seal, label, and date. Keep in the fridge.

You can take a teaspoonful of the strained liquid as needed.

VARIATION Try adding some chopped fresh thyme or sage to the onion.

SHELF LIFE Up to 6 months in the fridge.

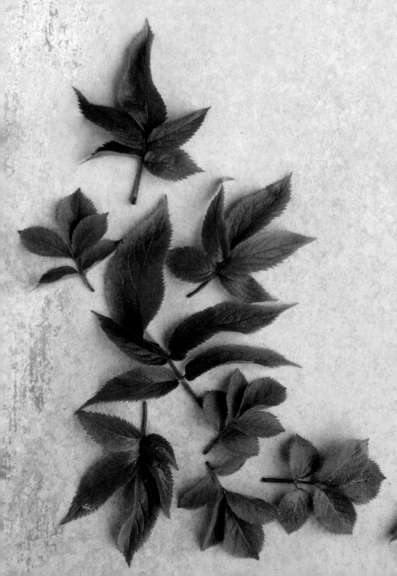

ELDERFLOWER, LEMON, AND GINGER COUGH DROPS

These antiviral cough drops help to soothe sore throats and ease coughs.

2-inch piece of fresh ginger, sliced
1 tablespoon whole cloves
5 fresh elderflower heads, main green stalks removed
    (or ¼ cup dried elderflowers)
elderflower cordial (optional)
2 cups unrefined sugar
1 cup honey
juice of ½ lemon
powdered sugar, to dust or for covering (see method)

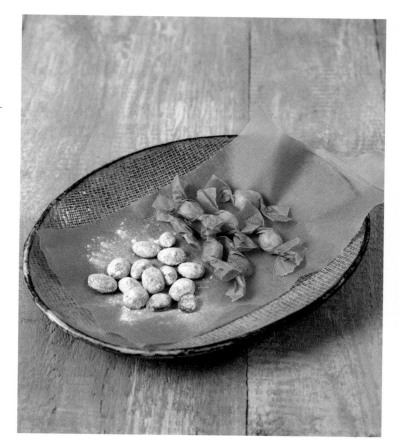

You will need to use a large, heavy-bottomed saucepan for this recipe (and select one that is about three times bigger in volume than the liquid you are using), otherwise the mixture will boil over.

Put the ginger and cloves into the saucepan, then pour over 1¼ cups water. Bring gently to a boil, then simmer, covered, for 10 minutes.

Remove from the heat, add the fresh or dried elderflowers, then set aside to infuse for 20 minutes.

Strain the liquid into a heatproof pitcher and measure it—you'll need 1 cup of the infusion for this recipe (if it needs topping up, then use water or elderflower cordial for extra flavor). Return the liquid back to the pan and then add the sugar, honey, and lemon juice.

Carefully heat until the mixture has come to a gentle rolling boil. Continue boiling gently until the sugar reaches the hard-crack stage (295–310°F on a candy thermometer), about 15–20 minutes. Caution, this mixture is extremely hot. This is the point at which a drop of the liquid will turn to brittle strands when dropped into a bowl of chilled water.

Once you have reached hard-crack stage, take off the heat. You can make your cough drops in one of two ways:

Drop teaspoonfuls onto a baking sheet lined with wax paper and leave to set, then sprinkle with powdered sugar after they have hardened to prevent them from sticking together.

Alternatively, take a baking sheet and fill it 1 inch deep with powdered sugar. Take an object that is the shape of a cough drop (the bottom of a cork works well here) and press into the powdered sugar to make lots of "molds," leaving a small gap between each one. Do not press all the way through to the sheet. Carefully pour a little of the sugar mixture into these indentations and then leave to set. Once set, remove from the powdered sugar, making sure the drops are coated all over (the powdered sugar can be reused, or see storage below).

To use, suck one sweet as needed.

To store, either wrap the sweets individually in wax paper and store in an airtight container, or store them covered in a thick layer of powdered sugar in an airtight container.

SHELF LIFE Up to 1 year in a cool, dark place.

ANTI-ALLERGY TEA

This refreshing tea is a traditional mix for reducing the symptoms of hay fever and allergic rhinitis.

2 ounces dried nettle leaf
2 ounces dried plantain leaf
2 ounces dried elderflowers

Mix all the herbs together in an airtight container, then seal, label, and date.

Use 1 teaspoon of the dried herb mix per 1 cup of boiling water to make an infusion. Strain and drink hot or chilled.

TIP Use fresh herbs when they're in season.

SHELF LIFE The dried herb mix will keep in a cool, dark place for up to 1 year.

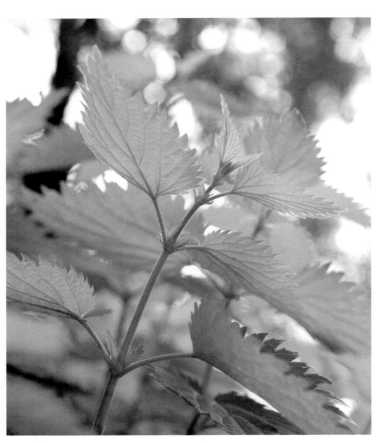

HAY FEVER

Hay fever can ruin a beautiful summer's day for sensitive people. A pollen allergy causes a range of symptoms including itchy eyes, congestion, sneezing, and coughing. Ideally start treating hay fever well before summer, to get your body ready for the season.

A very effective, tried-and-tested traditional mix includes elderflower, nettle, and plantain (see the Anti-Allergy Tea on the left). These herbs have an antihistamine effect, which helps calm the immune response and tone up the mucous membranes, drying up runny mucus. If you suffer from itchy eyes, a traditional addition to this infusion is eyebright.

Take the infusion at least once daily, and during the hay fever season take it up to three times a day. On warm days, take your tea served with ice and lemon and use local honey or elderflower cordial to sweeten, or make ice pops, which even children will love (see Anti-Allergy Ice Pops recipe on page 87).

HERBS *Nettle, Plantain, Elderflower, Yarrow*

COLDS AND FLU

Cold and flu viruses are common, particularly when the body is under stress. They can be the body's way of telling us to slow down and take some time to nourish our system. People often reach for symptom-suppressing acetaminophen and caffeine products at the first sign of a cold, to allow them to power through and carry on with work as usual. However, not taking time out to rest and heal can further weaken the body and prolong a cold. Acetaminophen brings down a high temperature, which is useful when fever is dangerously high. Many herbs act in a similar way; these are known as diaphoretics. They open the pores and encourage sweating, working with the body to gently bring down high fever. These include elderflower, yarrow, and linden blossom. During any kind of infection, viral or bacterial, we must also support the immune system (see Immune section on pages 56–59) with nourishing foods, vitamins, and herbs, such as echinacea and elderberry.

The first step to treating a cold would be to follow the old adage that "sleep is the best cure," so go to bed and sweat it out! Rest is vital for the body to repair itself and ensures it can concentrate on doing its job.

There is evidence that taking high doses of vitamin C (1000 mg) with zinc (15 mg) can help to reduce the length of a cold or flu. It appears particularly beneficial for those under physical or emotional stress.

Chicken bone broth—studies have shown that your grandmother was right: chicken soup is good for you. The nutrients in the bones of chicken help your body fight off infection and act in an anti-inflammatory way on an overburdened respiratory tract. Add raw minced garlic to the broth for an extra immune-stimulating boost. See the Chicken Bone Broth on page 56.

HERBS *Elderflower, Elderberry, Peppermint, Yarrow, Linden blossom, Echinacea, Self-heal*

ASTHMA

Asthma is a chronic inflammatory disorder that causes spasm and restriction in the airways. It can be caused or made worse with allergies (particularly in children), infections, exercise, and pollution. Symptoms include difficulty breathing, wheezing, chest tightness, and coughing. Herbal protocols would look at the underlying cause before the symptoms.

Mild asthma symptoms can be treated with gentle herbs by calming the immune response and relaxing the airways. Herbalists use thyme to encourage relaxed breathing and as a mucolytic, helping break down mucus. Wild cherry bark acts as an antitussive, relaxing the airways, and can help with breathing problems at night. Soothing demulcent herbs such as licorice and marshmallow are also useful. Use these in syrups or infusions. An aromatic chest rub can help open the airways and relieve tired, spasmed muscles.

Asthma has the potential to be very serious. If someone is struggling to breathe and is not responding to their normal medication, call an ambulance. For herbal

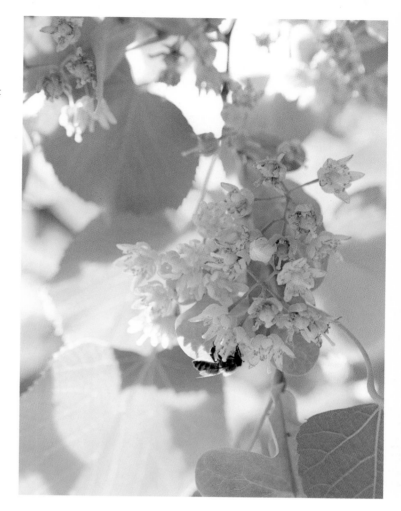

support for moderate to severe asthma, seek advice from a professional herbalist.

HERBS *Thyme, Wild Cherry bark, Honeysuckle, Licorice, Aniseed, Eucalyptus*

Linden *Tilia* spp. (above)
Nettle *Urtica dioica* (left)

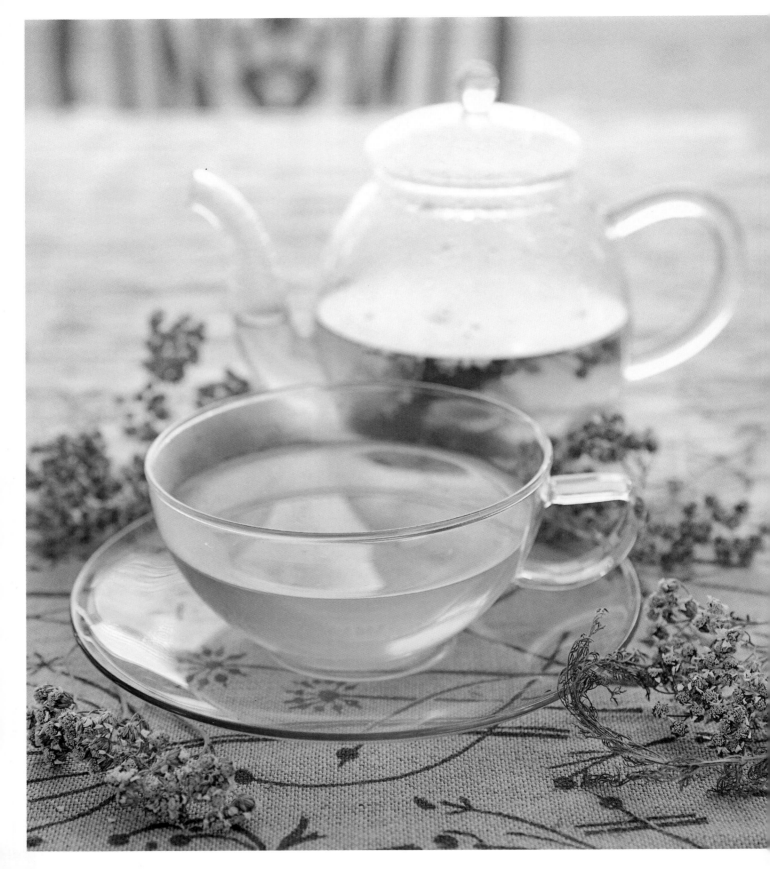

TRADITIONAL COLD AND FLU TEA

This antiviral herbal infusion is based on an age-old recipe. It combines astringent elderflower with anti-inflammatory yarrow and soothing peppermint to bring down high fever and decongest a stuffy head.

1 teaspoon dried elderflowers
1 teaspoon dried peppermint
1 teaspoon dried yarrow
2 cups boiling water

Place the dried herbs in a teapot or small saucepan, pour over the boiling water, then cover and leave to infuse for 15 minutes.

Strain, then drink a cupful when fever becomes high.

CHILDREN'S VERSION A simple infusion of linden blossom can be used for children's colds. Use 1 teaspoon per 1 cup of boiling water.

ASTHMA CHEST AND BACK RUB

This rub includes a combination of aromatic essential oils that encourages deep and relaxed breathing and eases tired muscles.

⅓ ounce beeswax
¾ cup olive oil
10 drops of thyme essential oil
10 drops of eucalyptus essential oil
10 drops of lavender essential oil
10 drops of frankincense essential oil

Dissolve the beeswax gently in the olive oil over a bain-marie.

Remove from the heat and leave to cool for a couple of minutes, then stir in the essential oils. Pour into a clean jar, leave to cool fully, then seal, label, and date.

To use, rub into chest and back, as needed.

SHELF LIFE Up to 1 year in a cool, dark place.

VEGAN VERSION Omit the beeswax and use ¾ cup coconut oil or shea butter instead of the olive oil. Melt gently in a bain-marie, then combine with the essential oils, jar, label, and date, as above.

COLD OR FLU?	COLD SYMPTOMS	INFLUENZA SYMPTOMS
Onset	Gradual	Sudden
Duration	Relatively short	Relatively long
Headache	Uncommon	Common
High fever	Uncommon	Common
Body aches and pains	Mild	Moderate-severe
Coughs	Mucus	Dry

THE URINARY SYSTEM

The urinary system consists of the kidneys, bladder, the tubes that connect them (ureters), and the urethra. It is an excretory organ system working alongside the liver, skin, lungs, and bowels to maintain the regulation of optimum body conditions. The kidneys filter the blood, removing and reserving useful substances and excreting wastes in the form of urine. Besides eliminating wastes, the kidneys perform a vital role in the health of the body as a whole: through maintaining the homeostatic balance of water, electrolytes, calcium, red blood cells, and blood pressure, and producing and interacting with various hormones.

Herbal infusions are the best way to get the most out of urinary herbs. Many herbs, such as dandelion leaf, cleavers, and nettle, act as diuretics to encourage urination and "flush" out the whole urinary system. If you are prone to water retention or bladder infection, drinking a cup or two of a diuretic infusion daily can help to keep the urinary system healthy.

ACTIONS FOR THE URINARY SYSTEM Diuretic, astringent/anti-inflammatory, antimicrobial, demulcent, immune tonic.

CYSTITIS AND BLADDER INFECTIONS

Cystitis is a painful condition caused by inflammation of the bladder, resulting in pain or a heavy feeling in the lower abdomen, burning during urination, and an increased urge to pee even if the bladder is empty. It is usually caused by bacterial infection and is much more common in women as the urethra is shorter and more vulnerable to infection and irritation. Cystitis can be chronic or happen a single time; either way, it can be extremely painful.

Herbal actions for treating a bladder infection include diuretics—this may seem counterproductive because there is already an increased urge to urinate, but increasing urine flow is the body's way of flushing out bacteria. Thyme, juniper berries, and yarrow act as urinary antiseptics to kill off bacteria inside the bladder and reduce inflammation. Use immune-boosting herbs such as echinacea to help the body fight infection.

A glass of unsweetened cranberry juice or a cranberry supplement taken daily has been shown to prevent bladder infections and lessen their duration. Other methods to prevent cystitis include:

- Wipe front to back after going to the toilet
- Empty the bladder after sex
- Stay well hydrated
- Wear loose-fitting clothing made of natural fabric
- Avoid scented and synthetic self-care products coming into contact with the intimate area (bubble baths, deodorants, soaps)

A useful first aid solution for cystitis, if you do not have any herbs on hand, is to make an infusion from the silky threads inside the outer leaves of a corn cob; drink this in quantity throughout the day for a few days until symptoms ease.

CAUTION Bladder infections can spread to the kidneys, which can be very dangerous. If you experience any kidney or lower back pain or blood in the urine, or if urine infections are chronic, seek medical attention.

HERBS *Corn silk, Echinacea, Dandelion leaf, Juniper berries, Cleavers, Plantain, Marshmallow root and leaf, Berberis, Thyme, Yarrow, Elderflower, Linden blossom, Ground Ivy, Rosemary, Eucalyptus*

PROSTATE PROBLEMS

Benign enlargement of the prostate gland affects many men from middle age onward. The prostate gland sits just beneath the bladder surrounding the urethra. If it becomes enlarged it can restrict the flow of urine, causing an increased urge to urinate, dribbling, and urine infections.

The exact cause of prostate enlargement is unknown but it has been linked to hormonal changes that occur with aging. The two main herbs used to treat the prostate are saw palmetto and nettle root; you'll need to see an herbalist about using these herbs. Adaptogenic herbs that increase overall vitality, such as ginseng, can also be added to an herbal treatment plan.

Prostatitis is an acute inflammation of the prostate usually caused by bacteria; the symptoms are similar to cystitis and are treated herbally in much the same way.

HERBS *Saw Palmetto, Nettle root, Ginseng, Echinacea*

CAUTION Always see a medical practitioner for diagnosis if there are symptoms of an enlarged prostate, to rule out prostate cancer before treating at home with herbs.

HERBAL SITZ BATH

A sitz bath is a warm, shallow bath made with an infusion of soothing and healing herbs. It is used to treat inflammation and discomfort in the pelvic region. This recipe uses antimicrobial thyme and eucalyptus leaves, along with soothing calendula and lavender, for use in urinary infections and thrush.

a small handful of fresh or dried thyme
a small handful of fresh or dried lavender
a small handful of fresh or dried calendula
a small handful of fresh or dried eucalyptus leaf

Add all the herbs to a large saucepan, pour over 2 quarts boiling water, cover, and infuse for 10–15 minutes. Leave to cool slightly, then strain before adding all the liquid to a shallow bath.

Soak and relax while the healing herbs do their thing.

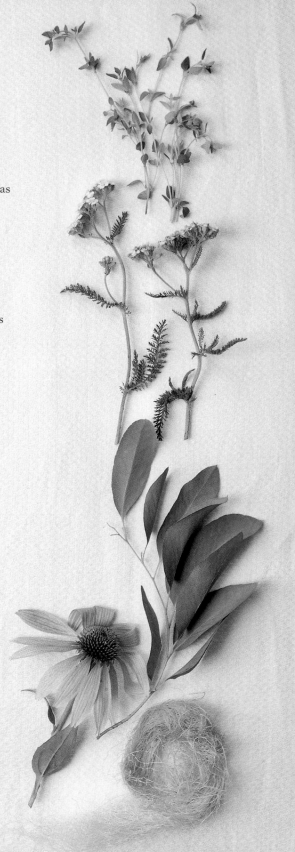

CHILDREN'S HEALTH

Children's immune systems are still developing, making them much more vulnerable to infection and allergies. Pair this with close contact to other children at school and day care and it can seem like they have constant coughs, colds, sniffles, and tummy bugs.

But this doesn't have to be the case. Just like adults, children can benefit from the right nutrition and a little herbal support. Herbs can be a safe and effective way to soothe and prevent illnesses in babies and children when used appropriately. The problem can be getting the herbs into them!

Children have more taste buds than adults and are programmed to prefer sweet and fatty foods. The bitterness of herbs can easily be disguised in infused honeys, syrups, glycerites, and even ice pops! Weak infusions or diluted drops of tinctures are usually quite well tolerated too, especially when mixed with some spiced Elderberry Syrup or Elderflower Cordial, or in Slippery Elm, Meadowsweet, and Milk Thistle Soothing Lozenges or Chewable Immune-Gut Gummies (see recipes on pages 141 and 48).

Get your children involved in the herbal "potion-making" process too. Take them outside and introduce them to nature's medicine chest, let them help to grow, harvest, and make their own remedies; they will be more likely to try them after putting in all that hard work.

When used correctly, herbs offer a safe and effective system of healing for the whole family. Many herbs are suitable for use in children provided they are given in the correct dosages; however, for home use it is best to stick to the gentle herbs listed here. These herbs can be used safely and regularly as part of your child's diet or daily routine. A pinch of antiviral thyme in soups and pasta sauces daily acts as a preventative during the cold season, or a cup of chamomile, lemon balm, and honey tea is ideal to soothe and relax them before bedtime.

When deciding how to administer herbs, bear in mind that dosages for herbal medicines are usually calculated for adults, so adjust the dose for the size and age of the child appropriately. Below is a rough guide for dosages for children at various ages.

DOSAGES FOR CHILDREN

When giving a new herb to your child for the first time, give a small dose and observe their symptoms/reaction to the herb carefully. As with dosages for adults, if treating an acute problem, it may be necessary to give small doses regularly. Whereas, if treating a long-term problem or preventatively, less regular doses taken 1–3 times daily is recommended. Below is a rough guide for dosages at different ages.

Babies 6 months–2 years: 10 percent of adult dose (consult an herbalist first for children under 2 years old)
Children age 2–6 years: 10–30 percent of adult dose
Children age 6–10 years: 30–50 percent of adult dose
Children age 10–14 years: 50–80 percent adult dose
Children age 14+ years: 80–100 percent of adult dose

HERBS SUITABLE FOR CHILDREN *Chamomile, Echinacea, Elderflower, Elderberry, Rose, Lavender, Linden blossom, Hawthorn, Peppermint, Plantain, Lemon Balm, Oats, Daisy, Cleavers, Calendula, Mullein, Honeysuckle, Poppy, Dandelion, Nettle, Violet, Wild Cherry, Selfheal, Chickweed, Marshmallow, Elecampane, Culinary herbs (see pages 154–165).*

ALLERGIES

There are thousands of possible allergens out there and different allergies produce a wide range of symptoms. The two most common allergies for children are eczema and asthma. Although these two conditions present quite differently, the core essence of treatment is the same; give herbs internally that allay the allergic response. An Anti-Allergy Tea (see page 80) combining nettle, elderflower, and plantain drunk regularly can help lessen the body's reaction. Childhood eczema can also be treated externally in much the same way as adult eczema (see page 72 for more details).

HERBS *Nettle, Elderflower, Plantain Dandelion, Calendula, Cleavers*

ANTI-ALLERGY ICE POPS

These ice pops combine the anti-allergic effects of nettle, elderflower, and plantain with soothing, sweet honey. Great for allergies of all kinds.

2 tablespoons dried nettle leaf
2 tablespoons dried plantain leaf
1¼ cups boiling water
½ cup elderflower cordial
2 tablespoons local honey

Make a strong tea infusion of nettle and plantain—place the herbs in a bowl, pour over the boiling water, and leave to infuse for 15 minutes, then strain into a pitcher.

Stir in the elderflower cordial and honey. Pour this mixture into ice pop molds and leave until completely cold, then pop them into the freezer until frozen solid.

To use, eat one ice pop per day, as and when needed.

SHELF LIFE Up to 1 year in the freezer.

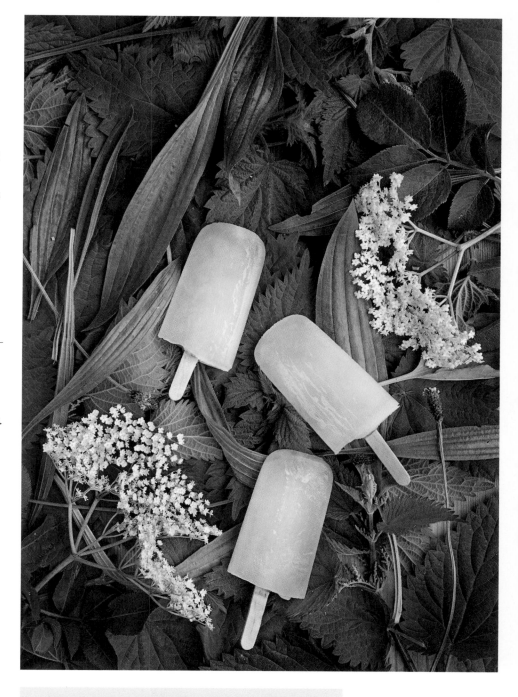

TIP Taking local honey internally is thought to desensitize the body's allergic response to pollen. Take a spoonful in a hot drink or enjoy an allergy-busting ice pop daily in the very early spring before the hay fever season starts, and see if you notice the difference.

CHICKENPOX

Caused by the varicella zoster virus, chickenpox presents as small, intensely itchy red spots all over the body. It is highly infectious among children and those who have not previously been infected. Symptoms tend to be mild in children but can cause general malaise, fever, and loss of appetite.

Chickenpox generally heals on its own, but you can support the immune system with elderberry and echinacea, alongside antiviral herbs such as thyme and lemon balm. An herbal cream applied to the "pox rash" can help calm inflammation and itching and prevent infection. Try the Soothing Skin Cream (see page 72) or, alternatively, try the Chickweed and Aloe Cooling Cubes (see page 144).

CAUTION If severe fever or headaches develop, see a medical practitioner.

HERBS *Elderberry, Echinacea, Thyme, Lemon Balm, Calendula, Chickweed, Oats*

COLIC

Colic in infants is characterized by long periods of crying in an otherwise healthy child. It is usually caused by abdominal pain from trapped air, which is taken into the gut when feeding. Making sure that the baby latches onto the nipple or bottle properly is essential to prevent the swallowing of air with milk. If breastfeeding, herbs can be ingested by the nursing mother and passed through to the breast milk. If bottle-fed, a small amount of weak infusion of any of the herbs below can provide relief. In newborns, you can rub skin-temperature infusion onto the tummy. Colic tends to clear up spontaneously at around 4 months of age.

HERBS *Dill, Chamomile, Fennel*

COUGHS AND COLDS

Children tend to pick up lots of respiratory infections; there are hundreds of different cold viruses out there and they have not yet built up immunity to them. Boost your child's immune system with a healthy diet that includes a rainbow of vegetables and lots of vitamin C. Give infection-fighting herbs like echinacea at the first sign of a sniffle. The spiced Elderberry Syrup (see page 179) served hot or cold is a delicious way to get immune-boosting herbs into kids, as are the Chewable Immune-Gut Gummies (see page 48).

Some coughs are wet and some are dry (see Respiratory section on pages 76–83). For wet coughs, use expectorant herbs such as thyme and elecampane to encourage the removal of mucus. For dry coughs, soothe and calm inflamed tissues with mucilaginous herbs like marshmallow and licorice. For dry coughs that keep the child awake at night, try wild cherry bark syrup; it suppresses the cough reaction, allowing time for healing and a peaceful night's sleep.

HERBS *Echinacea, Thyme, Elderberry, Marshmallow, Oregano, Elecampane, Wild Cherry bark, Violet*

CRADLE CAP

Cradle cap usually affects babies, causing dry, dandruff-like skin on the scalp. It appears red and raised in scaly patches with a yellowish crust. It is a common condition that has no clear cause and usually clears on its own accord. A balm made with calendula-infused oil can be massaged into the scalp before bath time to soothe and moisturize.

EXTERNAL HERBS *Calendula-infused oil, Olive oil, Stellaria-infused oil, Plantain-infused oil*

VOMITING AND DIARRHEA

Like many infections, children are often more prone to tummy bugs. Close contact with other children, rolling around on floors, and sticking dirty fingers in their mouths can lead to gastric upset. A little bacteria is actually good for us, as it helps build resistance and strengthens the immune system. Sometimes, though, it can cause vomiting and diarrhea.

An infusion of blackberry leaves sweetened with honey is an effective astringent that tightens up inflamed tissues in the gut. It is important to treat the infection as well as the diarrhea itself. See the Digestive System on pages 44–49.

CAUTION For severe vomiting and diarrhea, especially in children, seek professional medical attention.

HERBS *Meadowsweet, Blackberry leaves, Raspberry leaves, Chamomile, Thyme, Oregano, Hawthorn, Elderberry, Echinacea*

EAR INFECTIONS

Infections of the middle ear are very common in childhood, with about one in four children experiencing an ear infection by the age of ten. In most cases, ear infections develop quickly, sometimes as a result of a sore throat or cold, and resolve themselves within a few days, but they can be very painful. A few drops of lavender oil diluted in a teaspoon of olive oil massaged behind the ear can relieve inflammation and congestion. Mullein-infused oil is a traditional remedy for earache; a cotton ball soaked with mullein oil, placed in the outer ear can help lessen pain and swelling. Immune-boosting herbs taken internally may shorten the duration and intensity of the infection.

CAUTION For prolonged or recurring ear infections, seek medical advice.

INTERNAL HERBS *Echinacea, Cleavers, Elderberry, Elderflower, Garlic*
EXTERNAL HERBS *Lavender essential oil, Olive oil, Mullein-infused oil*

FEVER

Body temperature can rise quite dramatically in children and is usually the body's response to infection: a high body temperature creates an inhospitable environment for bacteria and viruses. However, if a temperature becomes too high it can become dangerous. Diaphoretic herbs encourage the body to sweat and dilate the small blood capillaries near to the skin, allowing heat to escape and reducing fever. An infusion of any of the herbs listed below can help to bring down high temperatures.

CAUTION If a temperature continues for more than 12 hours or exceeds 102°F, seek medical advice.

HERBS *Yarrow, Linden blossom, Elderflower, Peppermint, Self-heal*

HEAD LICE

Head lice spread from child to child through close contact. They live in the hair and feed off blood drawn from the scalp, which can cause itching and discomfort. Regular combing and washing with antiparasitic herbal shampoos can dislodge and discourage them. To make your usual shampoo antiparasitic, simply add 10 drops of lavender, tea tree, eucalyptus, or rosemary essential oil to each wash. To treat an infestation, try the treatment below.

EXTERNAL HERBS *Lavender, Tea Tree, Eucalyptus, or Rosemary essential oils*

HEAD LICE TREATMENT

An all-natural, bug-busting head lice treatment made with essential oils.

¼ cup base oil (olive or coconut oil works well)
10–20 drops of essential oil (chosen from the list above)

Blend the base and essential oils together in a small bowl. Massage the mixture into dry hair and the scalp, brush it through, and then cover the hair with a swimming cap. Leave the oil on overnight. In the morning, brush through with a head lice comb and remove any lice (dead or alive!). Repeat this treatment daily (overnight) until there are no signs of head lice.

INSOMNIA

Bedtime can be stressful for children and parents alike. It is helpful to establish a bedtime routine and relaxing herbs can be incorporated into this. A traditional remedy for helping children to sleep is a linden blossom bath. Make a large infusion using 1–2 handfuls of the dried herb in 1 quart of boiling water. Leave to cool to blood temperature and then add to a bath. Try a variation with lavender and chamomile, as these add a beautiful scent. Over time your child will start to associate these smells with relaxation and sleep.

The Soothing Tea for Children (see below) has a light and floral flavor and contains herbs that relax the nervous system, aiding a peaceful night's sleep. You can also tempt them with the Kid's Herbal Hot Chocolate.

HERBS *Linden blossom, Chamomile, Lavender, Rose, Oats*

SOOTHING TEA FOR CHILDREN

When children get anxious or hyperactive, this tea can help to calm them down. This can be used before a long travel, school tests, or before bed to encourage a peaceful night's sleep.

1 teaspoon fresh or dried chamomile
1 teaspoon fresh or dried linden blossom
1 teaspoon vanilla extract
1¼ cups boiling water
1 teaspoon honey, to serve (optional)

Put the herbs and vanilla into a teapot, then pour over the boiling water and leave to steep for 5 minutes (the longer you leave it, the more bitter it becomes).

Strain and allow to cool slightly. Serve with or without the honey.

KID'S HERBAL HOT CHOCOLATE

What better way to get herbs into kids than in hot chocolate? This recipe uses linden blossom–infused honey to soothe and relax hyperactivity or anxiety before bed. Almond, oat, or dairy milk also contain chemical compounds, including tryptophan and melatonin, that help the body to relax and drift off to sleep.

1 cup almond, oat, or cow's milk
3 cardamom pods
½ teaspoon vanilla seeds (scraped from a pod)
    or vanilla extract (optional)
1 tablespoon cocoa powder
2–4 teaspoons linden blossom-infused honey
    (see page 19 for instructions on how to make this)

Put the milk, cardamom pods, and vanilla seeds or extract (if using) into a small saucepan and bring gently to a simmer, then simmer for 5–10 minutes.

Remove from the heat and fish out the cardamom pods. Place the cocoa powder in a mug and stir in just enough of the hot milk to make a paste, then slowly pour in the rest of the milk, stirring constantly.

Stir in the infused honey, then serve.

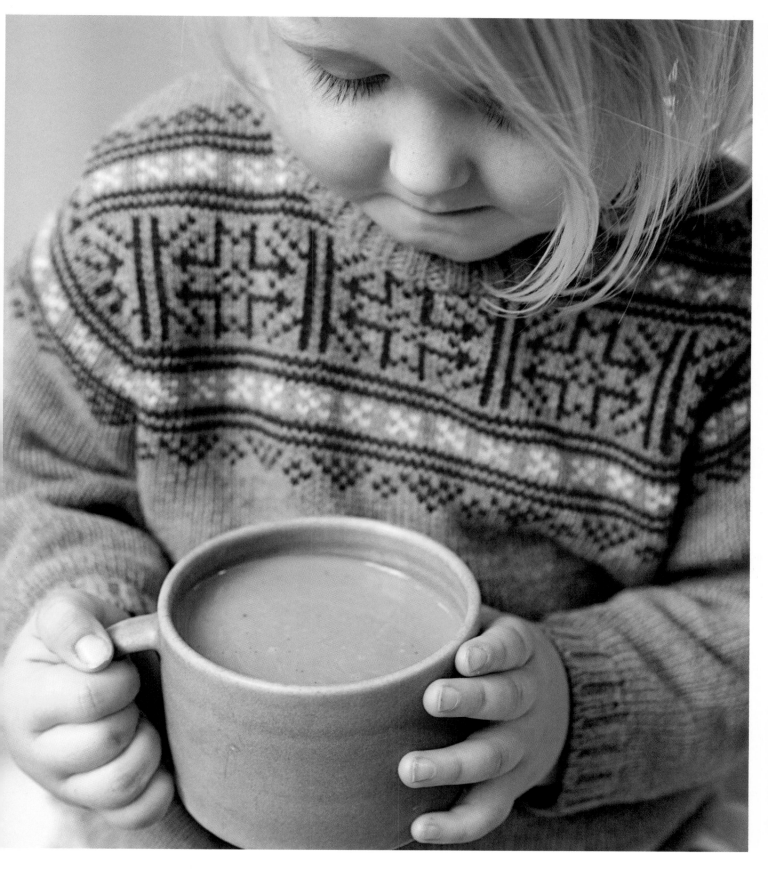

NAPPY RASH BARRIER CREAM

This cream contains soothing calendula, chamomile, and lavender to reduce inflammation and irritation. The zinc oxide or arrowroot powder acts as a physical barrier to protect skin from moisture and chafing.

⅔ cup coconut oil
a small handful of dried calendula petals
3½ ounces shea butter
¼ cup non-nano zinc oxide or ⅓ cup arrowroot powder
5 drops of lavender essential oil (optional)
5 drops of chamomile blue essential oil (optional)

Melt the coconut oil in a bain-marie, then add the calendula petals and allow the mixture to infuse over low heat for 30–60 minutes.

Strain out the petals and return the melted coconut oil to the bain-marie, then add the shea butter and stir until fully melted and combined.

Remove from the heat, then mix in the zinc oxide or arrowroot powder and essential oils (if using). Whisk well until cool. Spoon into jars, seal, label, and date.

To use, apply during diaper changing, as needed.

SHELF LIFE Up to 1 year in a cool, dark place.

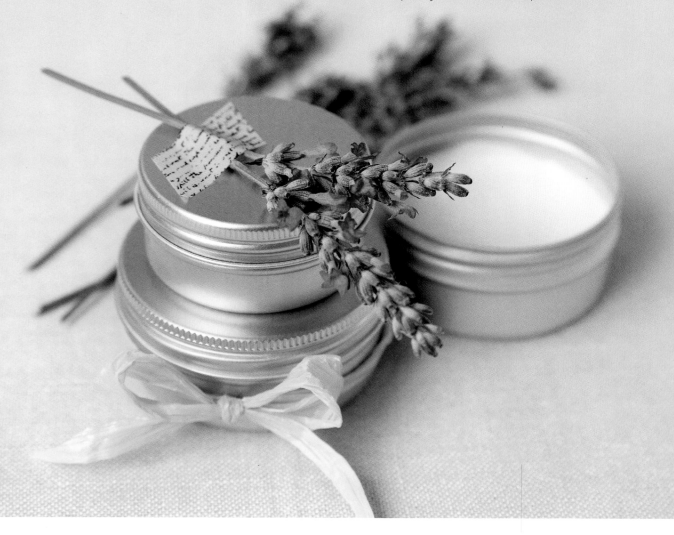

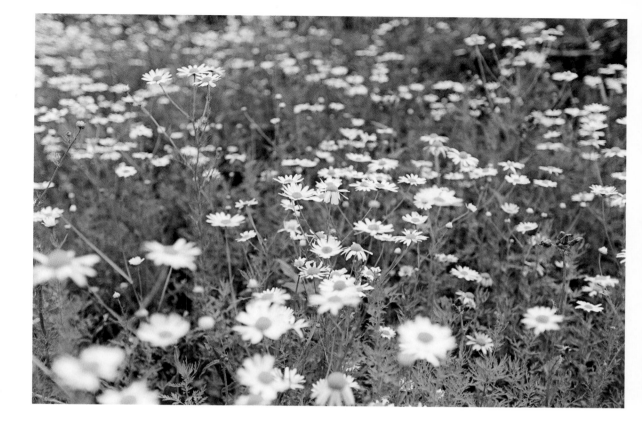

MUCUS AND CATARRH

Excessive mucus is the body's attempt to wash out a foreign body. It is extremely common in children as their immune systems are still being established, making them more prone to infection and allergies—the two main catarrh-causing culprits. If infection is suspected, immune-boosting herbs like elderberry and echinacea can be used. Elderflower and plantain are specific herbs for catarrh and sinus problems, especially where allergies are suspected—they gently tighten and tone mucous membranes. See the Anti-Allergy Tea recipe on page 80, or the anti-allergy infusion in the Anti-Allergy Ice Pops recipe on page 87.

Cut down on foods that encourage the production of mucus; these include milk, refined carbohydrates, and sugar. Replacing cow's milk with goat's milk or a fortified milk substitute can help to clear up chronic mucus.

HERBS *Nettle, Elderflower, Elderberry, Plantain, Echinacea*

Chamomile *Matricaria chamomilla* (above)

DIAPER RASH

Diaper rash is characterized by sore, red skin on the bottom caused by the moist environment of a diaper. Try to keep the area dry, allowing the child to go diaper-free when possible. An ointment made from calendula can help soothe irritation, or try the diaper rash barrier cream opposite.

EXTERNAL HERBS *Chamomile, Calendula, Stellaria, Lavender*

TEETHING

The cutting of first teeth in infants can be a stressful and uncomfortable time. To relieve pain, try soaking a clean cloth in a strong infusion of chamomile, then freeze for a soothing teething chew. A few drops of chamomile or calendula tincture, diluted 50:50 with water and rubbed on the gums, helps to numb pain and reduce the chances of infection. Diluted lavender essential oil rubbed onto the outer cheek can also help.

HERBS *Chamomile, Calendula, Lavender*

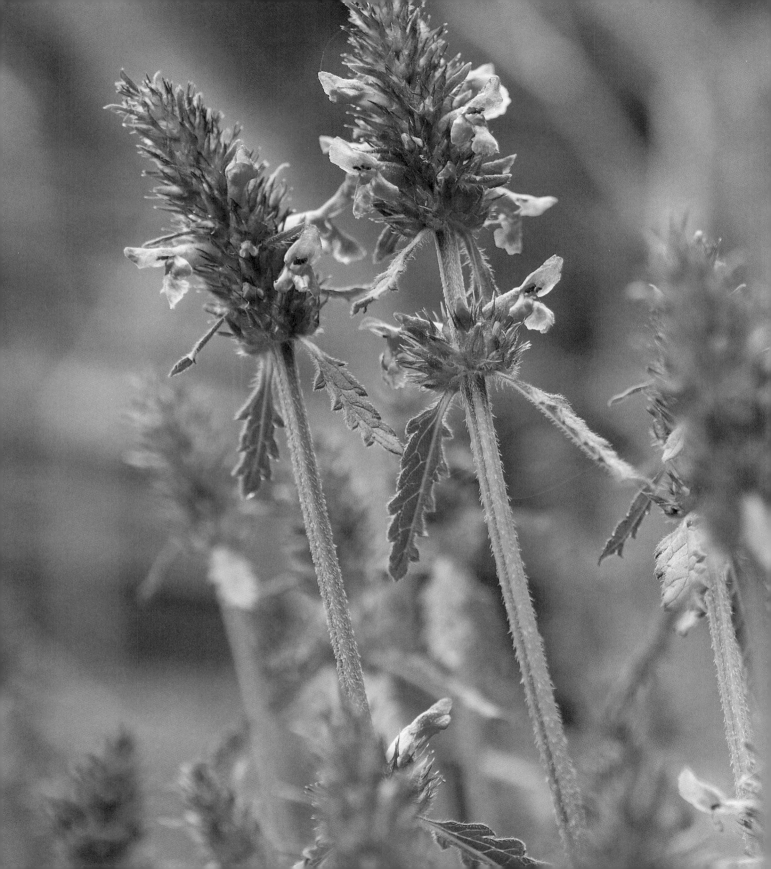

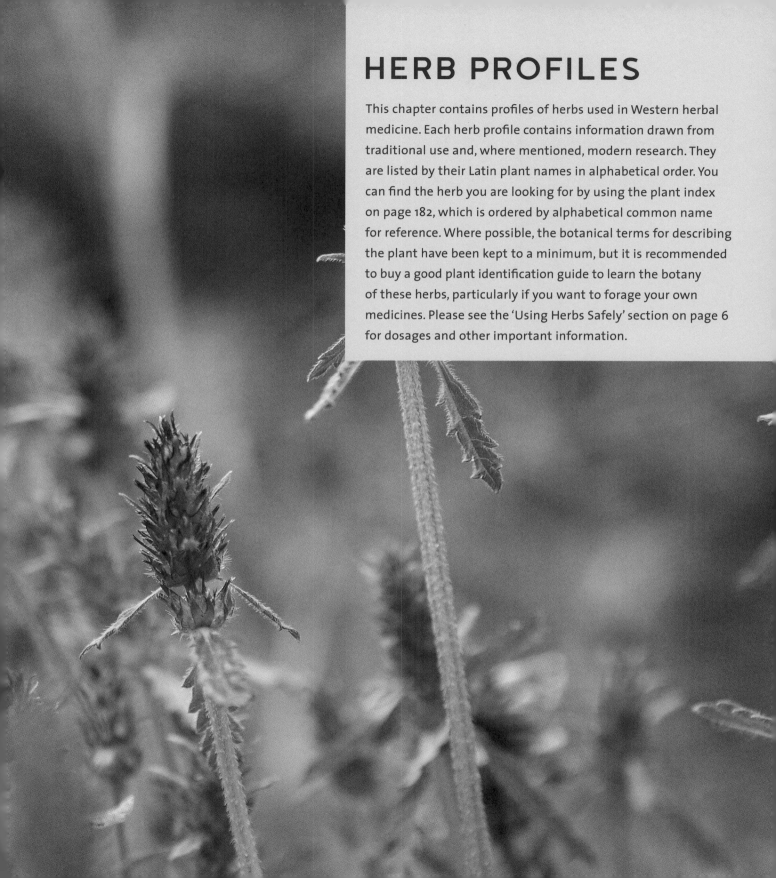

HERB PROFILES

This chapter contains profiles of herbs used in Western herbal medicine. Each herb profile contains information drawn from traditional use and, where mentioned, modern research. They are listed by their Latin plant names in alphabetical order. You can find the herb you are looking for by using the plant index on page 182, which is ordered by alphabetical common name for reference. Where possible, the botanical terms for describing the plant have been kept to a minimum, but it is recommended to buy a good plant identification guide to learn the botany of these herbs, particularly if you want to forage your own medicines. Please see the 'Using Herbs Safely' section on page 6 for dosages and other important information.

Achillea millefolium
Asteraceae

COMMON NAMES Yarrow, Nosebleed, Soldier's Woundwort, Milfoil

PARTS USED Flowers, leaves.

ACTIONS Astringent, circulatory tonic, styptic, anti-inflammatory, antispasmodic, bitter, urinary antiseptic, carminative, diaphoretic.

INDICATIONS Fever, high blood pressure, eczema, acne, rosacea, wound healing, hemorrhoids, varicose veins, heavy periods, scanty periods, spotting, period pain, endometriosis, fibroids, vaginal discharge, urine infections, digestive disorders.

DESCRIPTION Yarrow is a common weed that is native to the northern hemisphere where it can be found growing in meadows and fields. When cut or mown regularly it will stay small, leafy, flat against the ground and may never flower. When left to grow it can reach heights of up to 3 feet with whitish pink, aromatic flat clusters of flowers. Its Latin name, *millefolium*, means "a thousand leaves", referring to its feather-like leaves.

USES Yarrow is a powerful herb that acts specifically on the blood and circulatory system. Its gentle action means it can be used daily as a tonic herb to strengthen the circulatory system, making blood vessels strong and flexible. It possesses the ability to open up capillaries and allow blood to flow outward to the tiny veins in the peripherals, encouraging a stronger, larger network of blood vessels spread out through the system, which may help to lower blood pressure.

Yarrow has a normalizing, dual effect on the circulatory system; it encourages blood flow where it is lacking and also acts to suppress excessive blood loss. This normalizing effect is particularly useful in conditions of the female reproductive system, where it can regulate menstrual flow, break down clots and encourage the movement of stagnated blood. An infusion of yarrow taken daily is great for both heavy and scanty periods. By encouraging blood flow, it is also a great herb for period pain; if the uterus lining is shedding easily, the body does not need to cramp as much; therefore pain is reduced. Yarrow is helpful in any condition of the female reproductive system including fibroids, endometriosis and polycystic ovarian syndrome (PCOS).

A hot cup of yarrow tea is the go-to remedy for a fever; it lowers body temperature through opening up capillaries close to the skin, allowing heat to escape, "breaking" a fever. A traditional remedy for colds and flu is an infusion of yarrow, elderflower and peppermint.

For cuts and scrapes, a couple of clean leaves, chewed or crushed and applied to the wound, works brilliantly to help kill bacteria and stop bleeding in a first aid setting. An infused oil of yarrow is great to have in the medicine cabinet for wound healing of all kinds, as well as for hemorrhoids and varicose veins. A beautiful vivid blue essential oil high in the volatile oil azulene is extracted from yarrow; it is potently

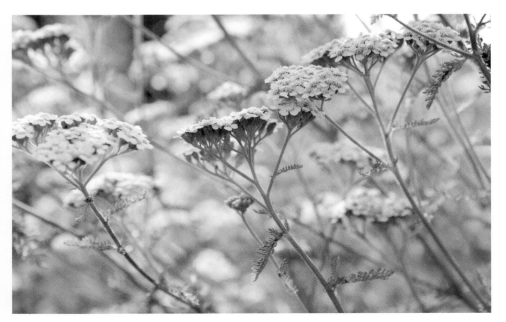

anti-inflammatory and great added to creams and lotions for use on eczema, rosacea, acne, and scarring.

For nosebleeds, the crushed leaves can be rolled into a nostril-shaped plug and placed in the nostril (not too far up!) until bleeding stops.

It is a slight diuretic and antiseptic and can be added to tea mixes for urine infections.

As it is an aromatic, bitter herb, yarrow encourages the flow of digestive juices, aiding digestion. Its anti-inflammatory effects also make it a useful addition for inflammatory gut conditions.

CAUTIONS Avoid in pregnancy due to possible uterine stimulating effects. Large internal doses may cause headaches. Prolonged external use may cause skin irritation in some.

Alchemilla vulgaris, A. mollis
Rosaceae

COMMON NAME Lady's Mantle

PARTS USED Flowers, leaves.

ACTIONS Astringent, styptic, emmenagogue, anti-inflammatory, vulnerary, menstrual regulator.

INDICATIONS Heavy periods, painful periods, irregular menstruation, spotting, diarrhea.

DESCRIPTION A beautiful perennial plant, its lobed, kidney-shaped leaves are borne on a basal rosette and covered in a layer of fine fuzz. Dew-like droplets collect at the base of each leaf. Medieval alchemists believed the dew to have magical properties, hence the plant's scientific name, *Alchemilla*. The tiny flowers are set in dense clusters and are yellow-green in color. *A. mollis* is a common garden variety and can be used interchangeably with *A. vulgaris*.

USES As the name suggests, lady's mantle's main use is in the treatment of women's ailments, where it helps

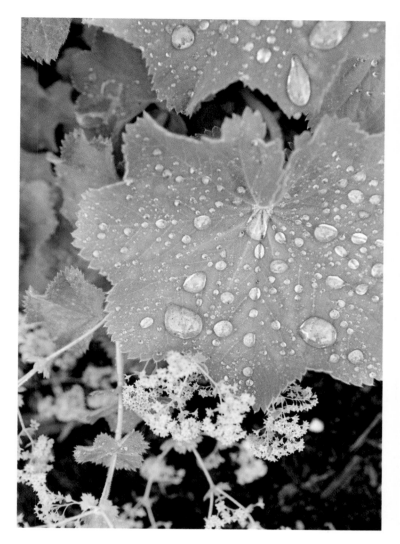

balance hormones and tone the reproductive organs. It is rich in tannins, making it a gentle astringent for use in the treatment of heavy menstruation, spotting, and painful periods. To get the most from lady's mantle, drink it daily as an infusion. For vaginal infections such as thrush, especially where there is discharge, lady's mantle infusion can be used as an external wash to soothe inflammation.

Traditionally, it was used in pregnancy to lessen morning sickness, prevent hemorrhage and miscarriage, and tone the uterus in preparation for childbirth. (Always seek a qualified practitioner before using herbs medicinally in pregnancy.)

Aloe vera
Asphodelaceae

COMMON NAME Aloe

PARTS USED Clear gel of the inner leaf.

ACTIONS Demulcent, soothing, cooling.

INDICATIONS Burns, sunburn, wounds, external inflammation.

DESCRIPTION This succulent plant can often be found in florists and garden centers. It has thick, fleshy, pointed green leaves flecked with white and edged with small spikes. When cut, a clear gel center is revealed.

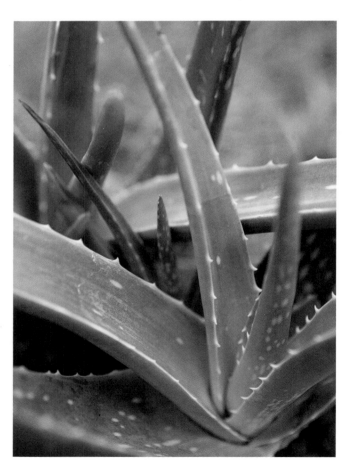

USES Aloe vera can be easily cultivated as a pot plant; it is a useful first aid herb for any home. The inner gel can be removed from the green parts by slicing off each side of the leaf. It can be used fresh for sunburn, burns, bites, and cuts, and adds an anti-inflammatory, cooling element to many healing and beauty creams; just use as part of the water component in a cream recipe. The leaves can be cut and stored in the freezer for future use; simply defrost as needed.

Traditionally, the yellow lining of the leaf was used as an irritant laxative but is no longer used as it is considered rather harsh, so take care to discard it when harvesting the aloe gel. See also the Chickweed and Aloe Cooling Cubes recipe on page 144, which is ideal for burns, sunburns, insect bites, and itchy spots and rashes.

ALOE BURNS CREAM

Aloe vera is an incredibly soothing and cooling remedy for burns and sunburn. Mixed with the skin-healing properties of St. John's wort and calendula, and pain-reducing, antiseptic lavender, this simple lotion provides a vacation and kitchen first aid essential. For this recipe, use pre-mixed (store-bought) aloe vera gel, which already contains emulsifiers to bind your cream.

½ cup aloe vera gel
1 tablespoon calendula-infused oil
1 tablespoon St John's wort-infused oil
20 drops of lavender essential oil

Place the aloe gel in a bowl and gradually whisk in the infused oils. Add the lavender essential oil and whisk again.

Place in a sterilized jar, then seal, label, and date.

Use liberally for burns and sunburns, as needed.

SHELF LIFE Up to 6 months in a cool, dark place.

Althaea officinalis; Malva sylvestris
Malvaceae

COMMON NAMES Marshmallow; Common Mallow

PARTS USED Flowers, leaves, roots.

ACTIONS Demulcent, mucilaginous, anti-inflammatory, diuretic, expectorant, astringent (leaves), emollient.

INDICATIONS Sore throats, cystitis, IBS, burns, rashes, boils, bites, gastritis, diarrhea, ulcers.

DESCRIPTION A tall and pretty perennial, growing to 5 feet in height. The leaves of *Althaea officinalis* are silvery in color and covered in a fine down, while those of *Malva sylvestris* are somewhat smoother and greener. The leaves of both species are roundish, 2–3 inches in length, and have 3–5 lobes. The flowers have five heart-shaped petals and range from very light pink to purple.

USES The whole mallow plant contains a gloopy mucilage when crushed, particularly the root of *A. officinalis*, which was once used in confectionery to make marshmallows. This mucilage component acts as a demulcent, coating and calming irritated mucous membranes throughout the body, soothing dry coughs, colds, gastric upsets, hot dry skin conditions and urinary infections.

Marshmallow is rarely found as a wild plant and so common mallow (*M. sylvestris*) can be used in its place; it is not quite as mucilaginous as marshmallow but is still a highly effective and more abundant alternative.

Mallow leaves are less mucilaginous than the root but are still demulcent. They are also slightly astringent. For external use on rashes, boils, bites, and stings they can be boiled in water for 5 minutes, left to cool, and then laid over the skin irritation. The leaves and flowers can also be mashed up and applied as a fresh poultice. Harvest the leaves just before the flowers form, and the root in late summer or early autumn. The whole plant is more mucilaginous when used fresh but can be dried for use throughout the seasons.

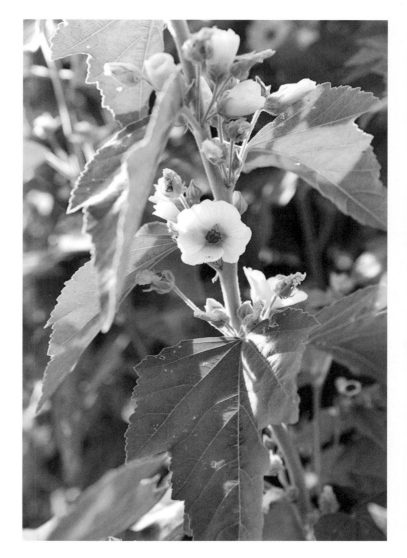

A hot or cold infusion made from the roots of mallow is mucilaginous, and can be applied as a compress for hot, inflamed rashes and sunburns. This can also be drunk as a tea to soothe ulcers, gastric upsets, coughs, and sore throats. Do bear in mind that small doses are soothing to the digestive system and can lessen diarrhea, but large quantities can be laxative. Marshmallow is so good at coating the tissues that it may lessen the absorption of other drugs and foods, so if using it internally, take it an hour or two before eating or using other medicines.

Angelica archangelica, Angelica sylvestris
Apiaceae

COMMON NAME Angelica

PARTS USED First year roots.

ACTIONS Carminative, expectorant, diaphoretic, circulatory.

INDICATIONS Digestive upsets, respiratory infections, urinary infections, menstrual problems.

DESCRIPTION Angelica is a biennial plant that loves to grow by water. It is cultivated for its roots, which can be increased in size by cutting back the first flowers. As with all plants of this family, make sure you know your identification, as there are some deadly relatives around.

USES Angelica is an edible plant — the stems are candied to create the green diamond-shaped sweets seen on old-fashioned cakes and the young leaves are tasty added to salads. It is an aromatic bitter plant, best paired with an added sour taste such as lemon juice. Medicinally, it has a wide range of uses; as a digestive tonic, for colds and flu, an expectorant in chest infections, as a urinary antiseptic, and as a menstrual tonic.

The roots contain an essential oil, which acts as a carminative for easing stomach pains associated with flatulence, and is included in many pre- and post-dinner, aperitif and digestif drinks around the world. It can be used in this way as a root decoction or a tincture and taken before or after food to help digestion.

Traditionally, it has also been used as an expectorant in cases of chest infections and for breaking fevers in illnesses, such as colds and flu, because of its diaphoretic properties.

Nibbling the root causes the mouth to go numb and tingle. This points to its analgesic properties. It also stimulates the circulation to the pelvic area, which might explain its traditional use for painful menstruation. Chewing a bit of the fresh or dried root can help ease cramps, or add to a decoction or tincture mix. However, angelica can increase menstrual bleeding in some people.

CAUTION Avoid in pregnancy.

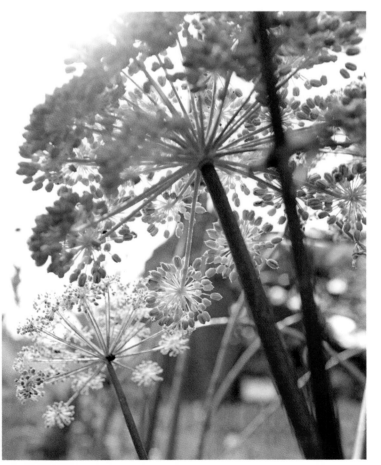

Arctium lappa
Asteraceae

COMMON NAME Burdock

PARTS USED Root, leaf, stems.

ACTIONS Alterative, diuretic, bitter.

INDICATIONS Digestive disorders, skin disorders, eczema, acne, psoriasis, infection, arthritis, joint inflammation.

DESCRIPTION This is a tall plant with evenly placed side shoots that give it an architecturally pleasing appearance. The leaves are a light to medium matt, dusty green with paler undersides. They are large enough to wear as a sunhat, one of its old country uses!

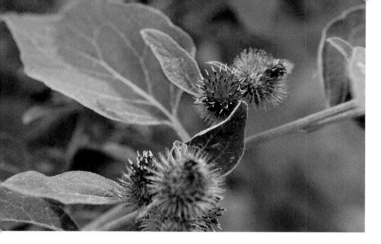

The plant is biennial; the leaves that appear in the first year build up food stores in the root; it then produces flowers and seeds in the second year. The roots are harvested after the first summer, before the next season when all of the goodness stored in the roots goes toward making flowers and seeds. The seed heads are covered in hooks that attach to clothes and animal fur as a method of seed dispersal. These hooks inspired the invention of Velcro, and along with the tiny hairs surrounding the seeds, make them tricky to harvest — gloves are recommended!

USES The stems and root of burdock are edible, and are eaten as a vegetable in many East Asian cuisines.

Burdock is bitter and is a primary herb for digestive disorders, particularly if the appetite needs stimulating or there is inadequate absorption of fats and/or nutrients and poor blood sugar control. It is also used in allergic conditions and dry, scaly skin disorders including eczema and psoriasis. Traditionally, the seeds were used for acute flare-ups and the root for long-term chronic conditions.

Dandelion and burdock syrup has been used since the Middle Ages. This digestive and diuretic action helps to support the liver and kidneys to eliminate wastes and clear skin and joint disorders.

DANDELION AND BURDOCK CORDIAL

A tasty traditional spring tonic to stimulate digestion.

5 ounces fresh burdock root
1 3/4 ounces fresh dandelion root
2 inches fresh ginger, sliced
2 quarts filtered water
3 1/2 to 4 1/2 pounds unrefined sugar

Put the roots, ginger and water into a saucepan, bring to a boil, then reduce the heat, cover and simmer for 30 minutes.

Strain the liquid and measure it into a clean saucepan, then for every 1 cup of liquid, add 1 cup of sugar. Heat gently, stirring until the sugar has dissolved, then simmer, stirring occasionally, until the consistency thickens, about 10–15 minutes. Pour into sterilized bottles, seal, label and date.

To use, dilute with cold water to taste and drink like a cordial.

SHELF LIFE Keep (unopened) in a cool, dark place for up to 1 year. Once opened, store in the fridge and use within 2 months (discard if moldy).

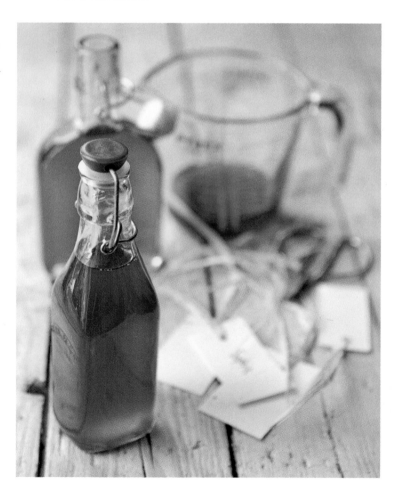

Artemisia vulgaris
Asteraceae

COMMON NAME Mugwort

PARTS USED Flowering tops, leaves.

ACTIONS Emmenagogue, nervine, bitter, digestive, carminative, anti-parasitic.

INDICATIONS Irregular cycles, painful periods, PMS, depression, anxiety, dreaming, poor digestion, lack of appetite.

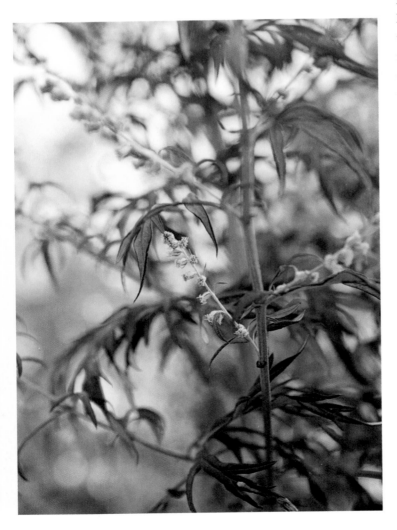

DESCRIPTION A tall and elegant plant, reaching up to 6 feet in height. Mugwort has pinnately lobed, deep green leaves, with silvery undersides; this feature distinguishes it from other *Artemisia* species. The flowers are small, silvery green, and borne in clusters.

USES Mugwort is an ancient herb enshrined in mystery and folklore. Dedicated to the goddess Artemis, it has been used for protection, psychic powers, and dreaming for centuries. A pillow made from the dried aromatic plant is said to banish nightmares and bring the user lucid dreams. A talisman of mugwort was thought to protect people and homes from evil. While it may not ward off evil spirits, its high essential oil content does repel insects and moths from the home when hung in bunches around doorways and in cupboards. Mugwort tea was traditionally drunk on an empty stomach to prevent and dispel worms and parasites from the gut.

Its bitter and aromatic qualities are employed in various aperitifs, helping to prepare digestive juices and stimulate the appetite before a meal. Its volatile oil content gives it antispasmodic effects, which are of value where there is spasm in the gut from wind and overeating.

Mugwort, herb of Artemis — the patron of women — has a traditional use as a female reproductive tonic, regulating menstrual flow and cycles. It has a reputation for aligning the menstrual cycles with the moon and bringing on delayed menstruation. Its antispasmodic effects can also lessen painful periods.

Mugwort has an uplifting effect on the mood, helping to relieve tension and soothe frayed nerves. It helps to relax the nervous system and promote restful sleep.

CAUTIONS Avoid during pregnancy or if trying to conceive.

Avena sativa
Poaceae

COMMON NAMES Wild Oats, Oat Straw, Oat Seed, Rolled Oats

PARTS USED Green seed, stems (oat straw), rolled oats.

ACTIONS Demulcent, nervine, nutritive.

INDICATIONS Anxiety, stress, skin problems.

DESCRIPTION Wild oats look like a tall, feathery grass festooned with elegantly hanging paper lanterns. These "lanterns" are the flowers hidden within a green, striped papery case that blow in the breeze to help pollination. The tips extend distinctively into long threads. It is within these cases that the oval pointed seeds develop. Harvest the aerial parts just before the seeds ripen and are still green. Pressing a fingernail into the side indicates its readiness: a milky liquid should be expressed.

USES Oats are familiar to us in the form of rolled oats or oatmeal. Rolled oats produce a soothing, gloopy mucilage that is a useful treatment for many inflammatory disorders, from skin problems to digestive irritation.
It soothes skin rashes, including allergies and eczema, and is a particularly safe remedy for children.

Oats soothe the digestive tract when irritated from vomiting or ulcers and are very nourishing for people recovering from illnesses. Oats are high in calcium and are an ideal food for bone and tissue strengthening, so if you have had a break or a wound, add some to your diet.

Both rolled oats and wild oats are a specific remedy for the nervous system, calming and soothing exhausted and highly strung nerves, particularly if caused by illness or long-term stress. Because of this, some herbalists also use them as a tonic for flagging libido and this may be the source of the saying "sowing your wild oats"!

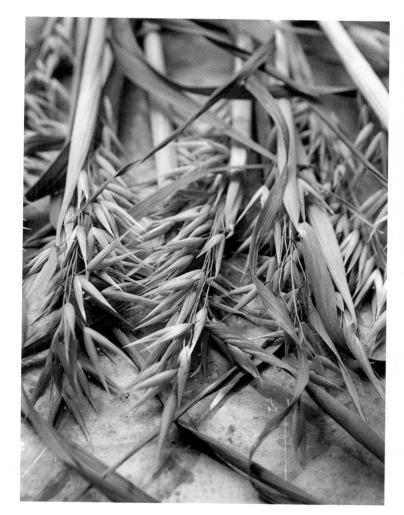

TIP For dry and itchy skin conditions, such as eczema, place a handful of rolled oats in a stocking or cheesecloth tied in a square. Use in the bath, like a soothing, milky sponge that comforts and moisturizes the skin.

Bellis perennis
Asteraceae

COMMON NAME Daisy

PARTS USED Flowers.

ACTIONS Anti-inflammatory, styptic.

INDICATIONS Bumps and bruises.

DESCRIPTION A small, perennial, creeping lawn and meadow flower. Slim white petals encircle a yellow button center. The leaves are oval and slightly fleshy. They can usually be found all year round in temperate climates but are most abundant in summer. The name daisy is a contraction of "day's eyes", referring to the fact that they open their petals during the day and close them when darkness falls.

USES A folklore saying affirms :when you can place your foot on 7 daisies, summer has arrived". It is the summertime daisy swathing many lawns, parks, and grasslands that can be identified with childhood pleasures. Many little children will have spent hours threading daisy

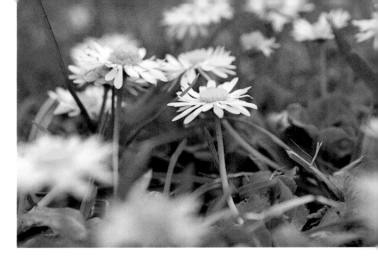

chain crowns to adorn heads. Their many white petals have also for time immemorial been a love "fortune teller"; plucking each one with "they love me, they love me not" foretells if your love is "true".

Despite being well known for childhood pastimes, the daisy has been medicinally overlooked in recent years. It was used as a salve for bruises, the sixteenth-century herbalist Gerard recorded it as "Bruisewort" – the suffix "wort" means a useful herb. This use can easily be harnessed for family first aid as a type of local arnica by infusing it in oil and turning it into a balm.

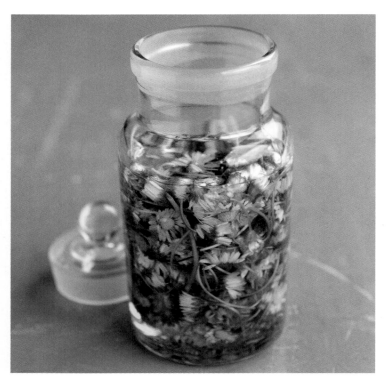

DAISY BRUISE BALM

This balm is ideal for bruises, bumps, and cuts.

a handful of fresh daisies
enough olive oil, to cover
beeswax

Take the clean, dry, freshly plucked daisy heads and place in a jar, then cover with oil. Cover and leave to infuse for a couple of weeks, after which time the mixture can be strained.

For every $\frac{1}{2}$ cup of strained oil, add $\frac{3}{4}$ ounce of beeswax and gently melt the two together over a bain-marie. When the beeswax has dissolved, pour the mix into a sterilized jar, then seal, label, and date.

To use, apply as needed. For external use only.

SHELF LIFE Up to 1 year in a cool, dark place.

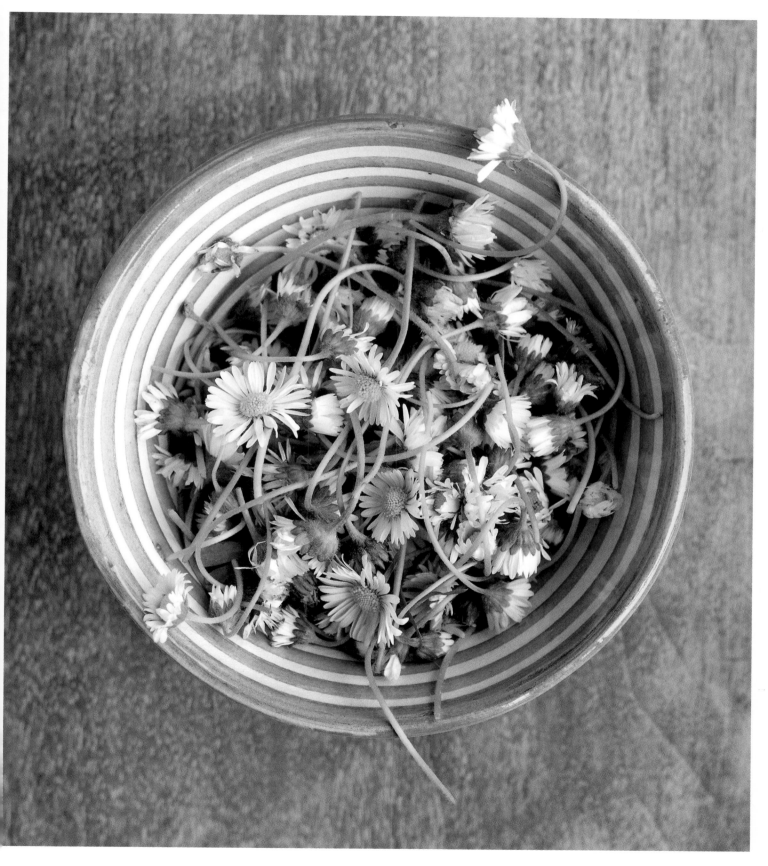

Berberis vulgaris (Berberis aquifolium syn. Mahonia aquifolium)
Berberidaceae

COMMON NAMES Barberry, Oregon Grape, Mahonia, Mountain Grape

PARTS USED Bark of root or stem, berries.

ACTIONS Bitter, alterative, laxative, antioxidant, antibacterial, astringent, liver tonic.

INDICATIONS Skin infections, acne, boils, eczema, wounds, poor digestion, diarrhea, gastritis, urine infections.

DESCRIPTION Berberis are deciduous shrubs commonly used as hedges. The leaves of *B. vulgaris* are small and oval with a serrated edge; *B. aquifolium* leaves are arranged on the stem like the ribs of an umbrella and are pinnate with oval spiny leaflets. Both bear small bright yellow flowers on clusters like spikes. The stems are woody and peeling the bark reveals a vivid yellow inner part. The berries of *B. vulgaris* are oval and bright red; *B aquifolium's* berries are a dusty purple.

USES Berberis species are used interchangeably in herbal medicine. It is the bark that is medicinal; the root bark is thought to have a stronger action than the stem bark, but they are both highly effective and the stem bark is much easier to harvest!

Berberis is an alterative, blood-cleansing herb; it aids in the clearance of bodily wastes, making it beneficial in the treatment of various skin conditions including acne, psoriasis, and eczema. Use the tincture or decoction over a period of at least 6 weeks to reap its full blood-cleansing effects. It can also be applied in creams and lotions topically for fungal skin infections and wounds.

Berberine, one of the alkaloids in berberis, has been shown to have anti-inflammatory actions and inhibit bacterial growth, supporting its traditional use as an anti-infective agent. Its bitter compounds stimulate the liver and digestion for the treatment of gastritis and general digestive debility. Its antibacterial effects can also be employed for the treatment of urine infections, sore throats, and respiratory infections.

The berries are produced in large bunches and are edible but sharp; when dried they make an interesting addition sprinkled over salads and rice. High in vitamin C and antioxidants, they also contain pectin and can be added to jam to help it set and give it tartness.

CAUTION Do not use in pregnancy.

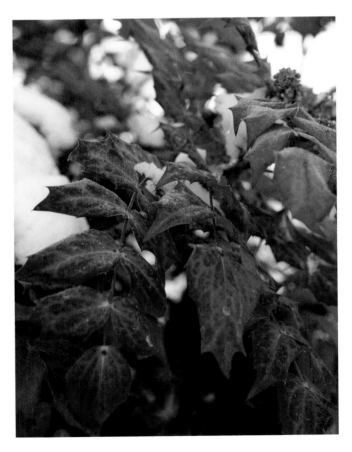

Calendula officinalis
Asteraceae

COMMON NAMES Calendula, Pot Marigold

PARTS USED Flowers.

ACTIONS Anti-inflammatory, lymphatic, antifungal, antimicrobial, emmenagogue, alterative.

INDICATIONS Inflammation, acne, eczema, infections, swollen lymph glands, bites, burns, wounds, painful periods.

DESCRIPTION Bright orange, daisy-like flowers characterize this herb, which blooms from early summer to late autumn in northern climates, after which it dies down and grows back from seed in spring. In warmer climates it may flower all year round. Leaves are alternate, oblong, and hairy. The whole plant is resinous and feels slightly sticky to the touch.

USES Calendula is high in anti-inflammatory flavonoids, essential oils, and plant sterols and can be used in inflamed conditions of all kinds. It is antiseptic, antifungal, and tissue healing, making it a great herb to use externally for wounds, bites, and burns. Internally, it encourages lymphatic flow, helping to rid the body of toxins, so it's useful for infections and swollen glands. Its lymphatic action helps brighten the skin and aid in the clearance of a number of skin conditions including acne, eczema, psoriasis and cellulite.

Due to its alterative, blood-cleansing effect, calendula is often added to teas and tinctures for menstrual problems, especially those where there is stagnation of the blood, which may cause heavy bleeding and cramping.

The resins and essential oils in calendula are antifungal and can be used both internally as a tea and externally as a wash or sitz bath in the treatment of vaginal thrush. A strong infusion of calendula can be used as a mouthwash for oral thrush and mouth ulcers.

Calendula's golden flowers are edible. Pick the petals from the flower heads and add to salads. The petals have a slightly bitter taste, which activates the liver and aids in the digestion of fats, helping to heal an irritated gastric system.

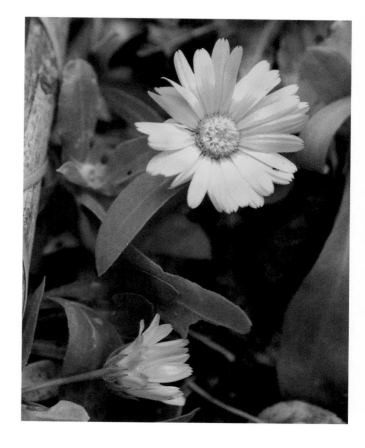

HEALING ULCER MOUTHWASH

This tincture and essential oil mix helps to tone and heal mouth ulcers. Alternatively, make an infusion with the fresh herbs listed here and swill at least twice a day.

³/₄ cup calendula tincture
½ cup raspberry leaf tincture
¼ cup sage infusion
10 drops of eucalyptus essential oil
10 drops of lavender essential oil

Place all the ingredients in a sterilized bottle, seal, then shake to mix. Label and date.

Shake well before each use. Dilute 2 teaspoons of mouthwash in ¼ cup of water, swill for 1 minute, and then spit out the mixture. Use as needed.

SHELF LIFE Up to 2 years in a cool, dark place.

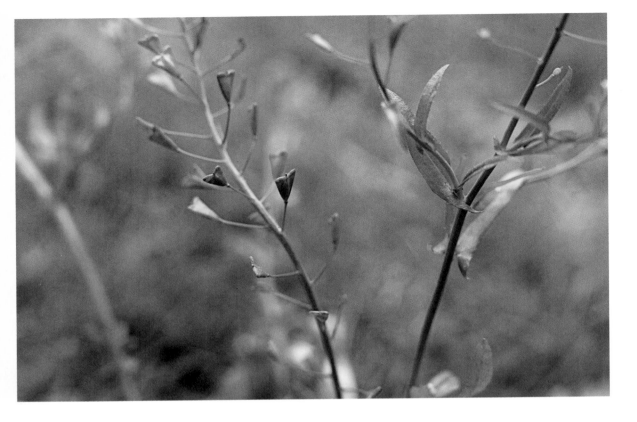

Capsella bursa-pastoris
Brassicaceae

COMMON NAME Shepherd's Purse

PARTS USED Aerial parts.

ACTIONS Styptic, urinary antiseptic, diuretic, anti-inflammatory.

INDICATIONS Heavy menstrual bleeding, diarrhea, wounds, cuts, urine infections.

DESCRIPTION A small unassuming herb that pops up in gardens, along roadsides and on wastelands. It has a basal rosette of deeply lobed leaves from which one or more flower stalks develop; the leaves on the flower stalks are much smaller and lanceolate-shaped. The flower spike produces small, white flowers, which go on to produce ladders of heart-shaped seed pods filled with tiny golden seeds, hence the common name shepherd's purse'.

USES This humble little weed is one of the most powerful herbs used to stop excessive bleeding, both internally for uterine bleeding and externally for wounds. Taken throughout the month it helps lighten heavy periods, lessen spotting between periods, and prevent flooding associated with endometriosis and menopause.

Because of its high tannin content, shepherd's purse tightens inflamed tissues, reducing diarrhea and soothing the urinary tract where there is irritation and infection. Shepherd's purse grows almost everywhere and makes a great first aid remedy for these problems.

Shepherd's purse is best used fresh, as it loses its potency quickly when dried. A fresh tincture is a good way to capture the plant's healing properties for later use. A fresh infusion can also be used but has a very peculiar taste.

Cichorium intybus
Asteraceae

COMMON NAME Chicory

PARTS USED Root, leaves.

ACTIONS Bitter, laxative, diuretic.

INDICATIONS Appetite stimulant, digestive tonic, anemia.

DESCRIPTION Chicory is a perennial plant native to Europe that has become naturalized in the United States, Australia, and China. It's related to dandelions, and can be found growing up to 3 feet high along roadsides and paths, where cars and people going by help to disperse the fluffy seeds. The flowers are multi-petaled and an unusual, beautiful pale blue.

USES Chicory root is commonly sold in health food stores as a caffeine-free coffee alternative and can be made at home by slicing, roasting and grinding the roots into a powder. Like its cousin dandelion, the leaves and roots are bitter and can be used in similar edible and medicinal ways, the effect being milder in action; the root of chicory is also bigger and easier to harvest. Chicory has a reputation for supporting the liver and kidneys. It was used in the past for flushing

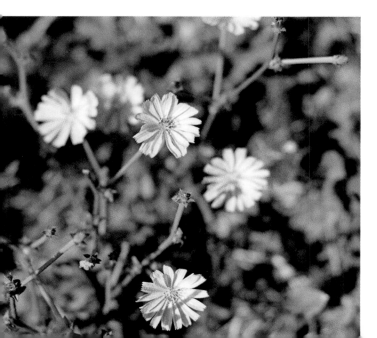

out crystals in gout and can be used to relieve joint pain.

Its bitter properties stimulate the appetite, increasing digestive enzymes and acids to increase nutrient absorption. This makes it useful for malabsorption problems and anemia. Though the taste is bitter, the leaves make a refreshing addition to salads or as a braised vegetable.

CAUTION Care should be taken with diabetics as it has been shown to lower blood sugar levels.

Echinacea angustifolia, E. purpurea
Asteraceae

COMMON NAMES Echinacea, Purple Cone Flower

PARTS USED Root, whole plant.

ACTIONS Anti-inflammatory, anti-infective, alterative, antiviral, immune modulator, lymphatic, wound healing.

INDICATIONS Infection, inflammation, swollen glands, acne, colds, low immune system, thrush, skin infections, post-viral fatigue.

DESCRIPTION Growing to around 3 feet tall, echinacea has purple to pink daisy-like flowers with prickly, cone-shaped centers, which give it the name, *echinacea*, meaning "hedgehog" in ancient Greek. It has a stout stem and deep green lanceolate leaves.

USES Echinacea is native to Northern America where it has long been used medicinally in the treatment of infections of all kinds. It is still arguably the most used herbal medicine in the world with various over-the-counter preparations available from health food stores and pharmacies alike.

Research backs up echinacea's immune-boosting and infection-fighting actions. Constituents found in echinacea, such as polysaccharides, isobutylamides, and caffeic acids, have been shown to support the body's immune response, reducing inflammation, increasing white blood cells, and aiding in the destruction and removal of unwanted bacteria, fungus, and viruses.

While antibiotics kill bacteria, echinacea encourages the body to make more immune cells, meaning that it can be used to support the body in both bacterial and viral infections. It also helps boost the immune system after prolonged illness in conditions such as post-viral fatigue, shortening the convalescence period.

One of echinacea's most famous uses is in the treatment of colds and flu. Studies have shown it can help reduce the duration of these, as well as lessen the incidence of respiratory infections. Take echinacea as soon as you feel a cold coming on to prevent it from becoming full blown. For sore throats, a tincture or decoction, used as a gargle and then swallowed, helps to numb pain and clear infection and inflammation. Alternatively, use the Echinacea Sore Throat Spray (see right).

Used internally and topically, echinacea helps to clear skin wounds, acne and infections such as ringworm, impetigo, and thrush. Make a paste from the root powder mixed with water, or use the diluted tincture on some clean gauze or cotton to bathe the affected area.

CAUTIONS May interact with immunosuppressant drugs. Seek professional advice when using in autoimmune conditions. Do not use in known sensitivity to the daisy (*Asteraceae*) family.

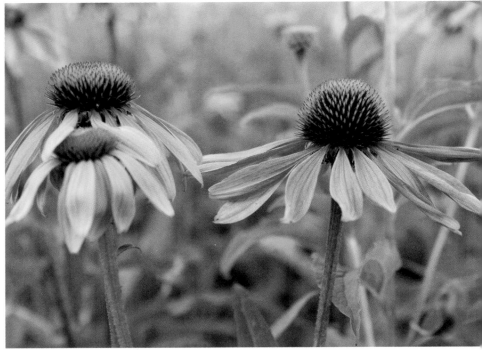

ECHINACEA SORE THROAT SPRAY

This spray contains echinacea, which stimulates the immune system and provides a fresh, tingling pain relief for a two-in-one action.

1 tablespoon elderberry infusion
2 teaspoons honey or glycerin
4 teaspoons echinacea tincture
1 teaspoon sage tincture

While the elderberry infusion is still warm, mix in the honey or glycerin to dissolve.

Pour into a sterilized 2 ounce (¼ cup) spray bottle, add the two tinctures and mix well. Seal, label, and date.

To use, spray onto the back of the throat, as needed.

SHELF LIFE Up to 1 year in a cool, dry place.

Equisetum arvense
Equisetaceae

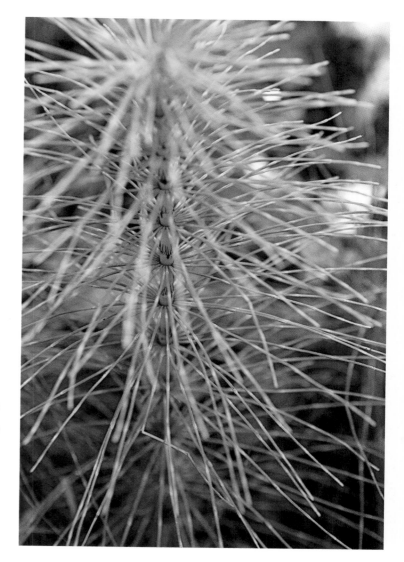

COMMON NAME Horsetail

PARTS USED Young leafy stems (not the first spore-producing, bare stems, but the later spiky-leafed ones).

ACTIONS Diuretic, nutritive, re-mineralizer.

INDICATIONS Broken bones, tissue strengthening, hair and nail strengthening, cystitis.

DESCRIPTION This is the last survivor in a family of prehistoric plants, and looking at it, you can see it is a strange, primitive-looking herb! There are many species of horsetails. It is named horsetail because the stem looks jointed like the bones from a horse's tail. Many species are used interchangeably around the world, but the main medicinal one is *E. arvense*; check with your local herbalist to see if others are used.

USES This plant has been mainly used for its high mineral content, particularly silica, and its effect on bone and tissue healing. It is used for strengthening weak and broken bones, pulled tendons and weak skin, hair, and nails. Though it isn't clear quite how it works, it seems to have an effect on the structure of bones similar to the way mortar holds bricks together. The high mineral content can be felt on the plant as the silica gives it a fine sandpaper feel, and because of this it has been used as a pot scrubber.

Traditionally, it is taken as a tea, tincture, or syrup. Juicing it is a good way to get the silica into your diet, though use sparingly for short periods and with demulcents like marshmallow to balance the dryness of the herb. Horsetail is also a diuretic used to flush out urinary infections.

CAUTIONS People with heart or kidney problems. Those with low vitamin B (horsetail contains an enzyme that can prevent adequate vitamin B use). Avoid in pregnancy. Take care when using old dried stems, as the particles can be irritating to the lungs if handled frequently.

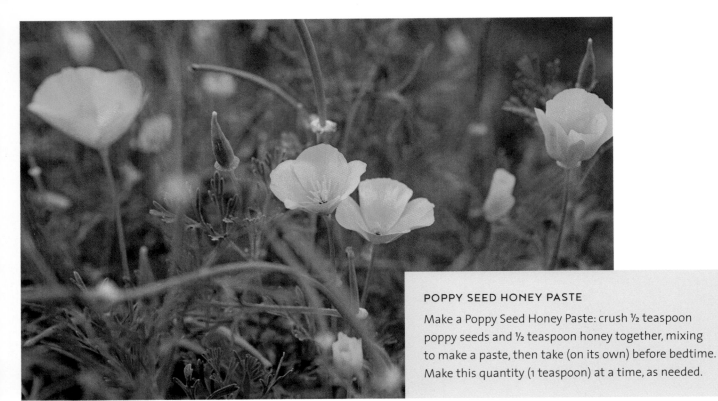

Eschscholzia californica; Papaver rhoeas
Papaveraceae

COMMON NAMES California Poppy, Golden Poppy, Corn Poppy, Red Poppy, Common Poppy, Flanders Poppy

PARTS USED Flowers, leaves, seeds.

ACTIONS Analgesic, antispasmodic, sedative, diaphoretic.

INDICATIONS Insomnia, nervous tension, headaches, dry coughs, pain, sciatica.

DESCRIPTION

CALIFORNIA POPPY A perennial plant growing up to 2 feet in height, with golden petals that range in color from yellow to orange (pictured above). The flowers close up into a pretty spiral trumpet shape at night and during cold or windy weather. California poppy flowers from very early spring to autumn. Seed pods are long and thin. Leaves are deeply lobed.

CORN POPPY An annual plant with large, bright red, delicate flowers growing to about 2 feet in height. Seeds form in smooth cups ½ to ³/₄ inch long that look like people wearing little hats. Leaves are deeply lobed.

USES Poppies come in many different shapes, colors, and sizes. The two main species used in herbal medicine today are California poppy and corn poppy. Both grow commonly as garden escapes, along roadsides, and in unkempt lawns and fields.

Both are used in much the same way medicinally: to relieve pain and induce sleep. Unlike their cousin the opium poppy, corn and California poppies do not contain addictive opiates. They do contain some opiates, but these are much gentler and are considered safe for use, even in children and the elderly, when used in the correct dosage.

The medicinal effects of these poppies come from various alkaloids present in the milky latex, which exudes from the fresh leaves and green seed pods when broken or crushed. The flowers and seed heads can be made into tinctures or dried into teas for use in insomnia and nervous tension. For a relaxing nighttime tea, combine with linden blossom and chamomile.

Poppy flowers work really well as a glycerite to soothe and suppress dry, irritated coughs. They reduce muscle spasm and relieve painful, tight rib muscles when excessive coughing causes them to become sore. Poppy encourages sweating and so is useful to break a fever, especially where there is pain involved.

The seeds of California poppy and corn poppy are edible and are delicious added to all kinds of dishes and cakes; they also possess sedative and pain-relieving effects.

CAUTION Avoid in pregnancy.

Filipendula ulmaria
Rosaceae

COMMON NAME Meadowsweet

PARTS USED Flowers, upper leaves.

ACTIONS Antirheumatic, anti-arthritic, painkilling, anti-inflammatory.

INDICATIONS Digestive disorders, arthritis, muscle and joint pain, general pain and inflammation.

DESCRIPTION Meadowsweet grows in damp places such as ditches and flood meadows. The name meadowsweet refers to its use as a sweetener for the alcoholic drink mead. The flowers grow in lush, creamy spikes, with a scent reminiscent of sweet almonds.

USES The glorious lush scent of meadowsweet made it popular in the past as a strewing herb — a fresh carpet of fragrant herbs placed on the floor to protect from dirt, scent rooms, and repel pests. The taste is as good as the smell and it is delicious made into a syrup (use the Elderflower Cordial recipe on page 180, replacing the elderflowers with fresh meadowsweet blooms).

Medicinally, meadowsweet is a specific remedy for problems of the digestive tract. It calms and cools heartburn and is a tonic for tummy upsets, nausea, post-vomiting, diarrhea recovery, and even hangovers. It is best for these conditions used in an infusion, or try the digestive Soothing Lozenges recipe on page 141.

The original name for meadowsweet was spirea, which is where the name aspirin came from. Though it was originally discovered in willow bark, the aspirin compound salicylic acid was subsequently extracted from meadowsweet. This salicylic acid content makes it a powerful anti-inflammatory and pain reliever for soothing arthritic conditions, and for inflamed and painful joints. It can be taken internally in teas and tinctures or as a warming bath for these problems. The flowers can also be used to infuse oil to make an external rub for soothing aches and pains.

CAUTION Not suitable for people sensitive to salicylates.

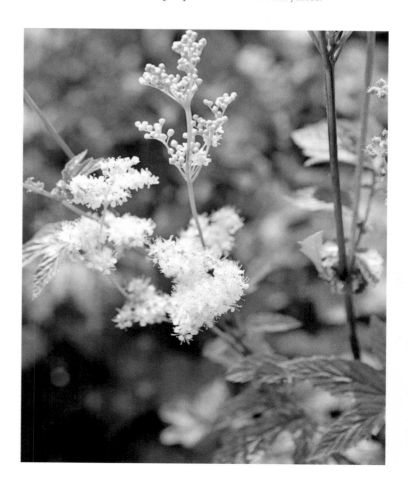

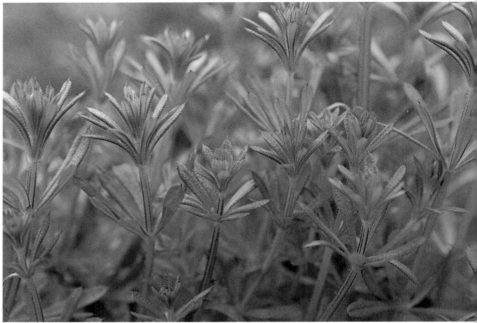

Galium aparine
Rubiaceae

COMMON NAMES Cleavers, Goosegrass, Sticky Willie, Sticky Weed

PARTS USED Whole fresh, aerial plant.

ACTIONS Anti-inflammatory, diuretic, alterative, lymphatic, tonic.

INDICATIONS Chronic skin conditions, acne, eczema, psoriasis, urticaria, infection, swollen lymph nodes, tonsillitis, cellulite, cystitis.

DESCRIPTION The lanky-looking cleavers plant sends up its bright green shoots in the early spring and is one of the first plants to sprout up in the herbal year. Its square-shaped, creeping stems can sprawl out up to 9 feet in all directions and are covered in whorls of 6–10 leaves, with tiny green-white star-shaped flowers. The whole plant is covered in Velcro-like sticky hairs, including the seeds, which stick to pets and ankles hoping to be spread far and wide, hence the name sticky weed.

USES Cleavers is a powerful yet gentle lymphatic, used in virtually any condition characterized by inflammation. Traditionally it was used as a blood-cleansing herb, aiding in the removal of metabolic wastes and helping to clear infections of any kind, bringing down swollen glands, adenoids, and tonsils.

It is invaluable in the treatment of skin conditions including eczema, acne, psoriasis, and slow-to-heal infections. It can help to brighten up the complexion, washing out bogged-down tissues. An old saying goes "whoever should only drink cleavers water for 9 weeks shall be so beautiful, everyone will fall in love with them." It contains high amounts of silica, an essential nutrient for maintaining hair, skin and nail growth and repair. Its affiliation with the lymphatic system makes it a great spring cleansing herb that can help to kick-start a sluggish system after a long winter of rich foods and hibernation. It also has a great reputation for reducing cellulite.

Cleavers acts as a diuretic, increasing urine flow, so helping to ease painful urinary tract infections and water retention.

The whole plant is highly nutritious and many foraging books and blogs recommend eating cleavers like spinach. While it has a beautifully fresh, crisp taste (a bit like cucumber mixed with new potatoes!), the texture is harsh, even when finely chopped and boiled (the tiny hairs can make it hard to swallow), so use it only when very young or sparingly in food.

Cleavers is best used fresh and should be harvested before it goes to seed in the summer. Use cleavers in a cold infusion (see opposite) or make fresh herb tinctures or juice and freeze for later use (see also the cleavers entry in the Wild Green Edibles section on page 26 for more details).

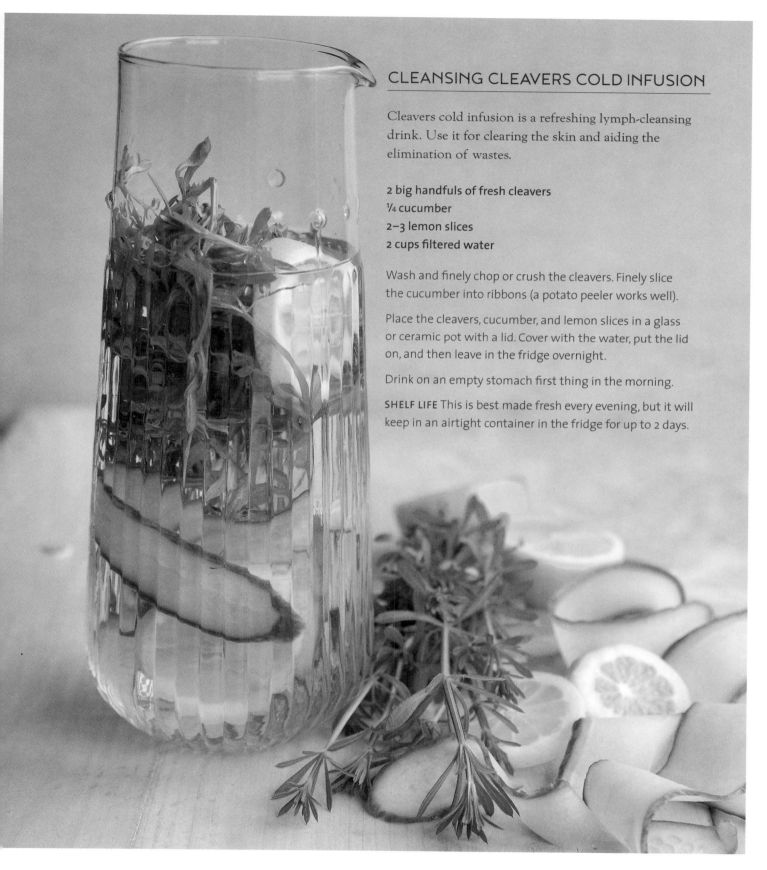

CLEANSING CLEAVERS COLD INFUSION

Cleavers cold infusion is a refreshing lymph-cleansing drink. Use it for clearing the skin and aiding the elimination of wastes.

2 big handfuls of fresh cleavers
¼ cucumber
2–3 lemon slices
2 cups filtered water

Wash and finely chop or crush the cleavers. Finely slice the cucumber into ribbons (a potato peeler works well).

Place the cleavers, cucumber, and lemon slices in a glass or ceramic pot with a lid. Cover with the water, put the lid on, and then leave in the fridge overnight.

Drink on an empty stomach first thing in the morning.

SHELF LIFE This is best made fresh every evening, but it will keep in an airtight container in the fridge for up to 2 days.

Geranium robertianum
Geraniaceae

COMMON NAMES Herb Robert, Cranesbill

PARTS USED Aerial parts.

ACTIONS Astringent, styptic, antiseptic.

INDICATIONS Skin infections, wounds, bruises, insect bites.

DESCRIPTION A small, hairy plant with deep green, highly lobed leaves and multiple juicy, red stems that arise in clusters from the same point. The flowers have five pinkish purple petals and seed pods that are pointed like cranes' bills.

USES Herb Robert has a rich history of use as a wound herb. In recent years, it has fallen out of popularity among herbalists for no apparent reason. Herb Robert's commonness makes it a perfect first aid herb, often found growing in between patio cracks and sprouting up in flowerbeds. Its availability throughout most of the year means it can be used fresh; simply crush and apply the juice to bruises, cuts and wounds — it encourages healing and prevents excess bleeding. It is specifically good for slow-to-heal wounds and where granulation (tissue growth) is needed.

Rolled up into a plug and placed into the nostril, herb Robert helps to stop nosebleeds, although it does have a very peculiar smell, somewhat like burning rubber! Its aroma comes in handy as an emergency bug repellent should you find yourself on the menu for mosquitoes. Simply rub the leaves over exposed skin.

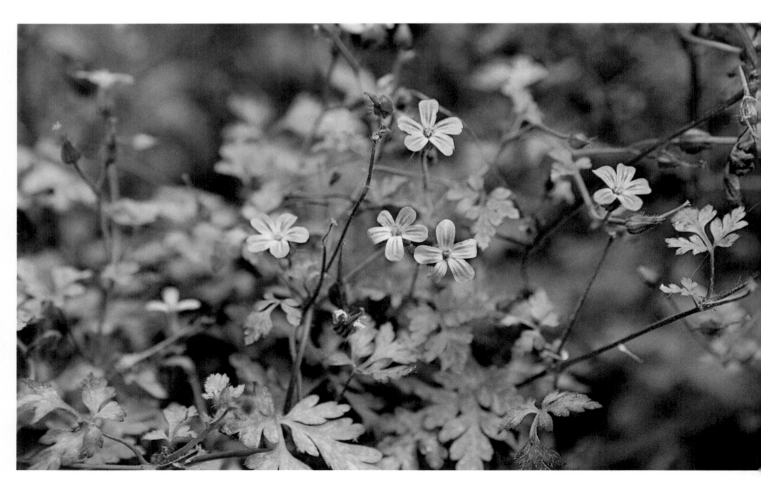

Glechoma hederacea
Lamiaceae

COMMON NAMES Ground Ivy

PARTS USED Aerial parts.

ACTIONS Bitter, expectorant, decongestant, diuretic, astringent, vulnerary.

INDICATIONS Sore throats, wounds, chest infections, bronchitis, sinusitis, urinary infections.

DESCRIPTION A perennial creeper of the mint family. Ground ivy's dark green leaves are opposite, hairy and kidney-shaped with a scalloped edge. Flowers are blue to violet in color and grow in clusters of 2–3 at the leaf axils. The young growing tips of the plant are often tinged with deep purple, making it an attractive ground cover plant in dark, damp corners of the garden.

USES Ground ivy has a long and respected history as a potent and multifaceted medicine. Unfortunately, it has fallen out of "health fashion" in recent years. It is common and often found growing in gardens and parks and can be used for a plethora of ailments, making it a very useful remedy.

Historically, ground ivy was used in conditions of the eyes and kidneys; today it is still a useful diuretic for the treatment of cystitis and bladder infections. It is a gentle, effective astringent, tightening and toning inflamed tissues, and was employed traditionally as a wound herb and for diarrhea. Used as a gargle, it soothes a sore throat and mouth ulcers. It is a specific remedy for sinusitis, reducing catarrh in the respiratory tract and acting as a decongestant for chest infections and bronchitis.

Ground ivy is edible and once was used as a salad herb; it has a distinct peppery flavor with a bitter quality to it that stimulates digestion. It has a high content of minerals and vitamin C and can be chopped finely and sprinkled over salads, or cooked in soups and casseroles. The flavor intensifies with age so it is best used while young.

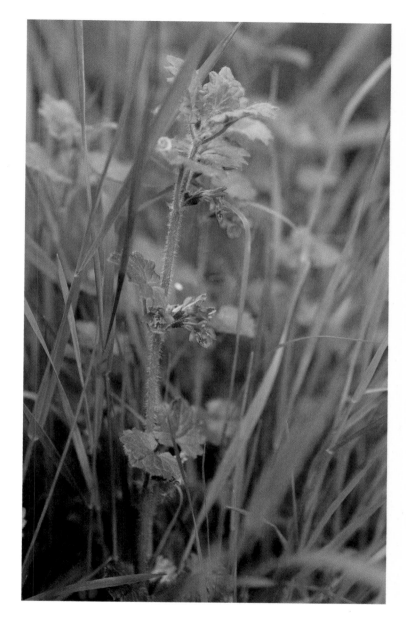

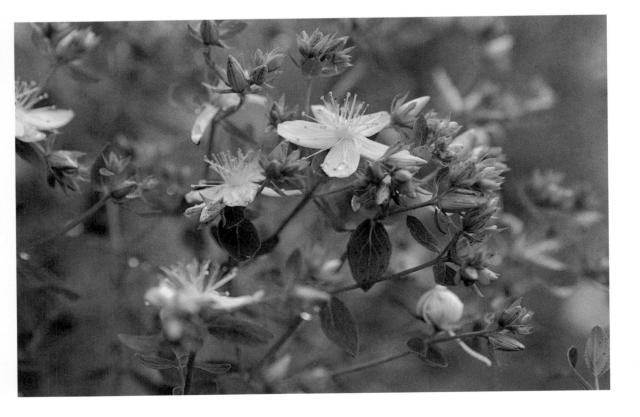

Hypericum perforatum
Hypericaceae

COMMON NAMES St. John's Wort, Klamath Weed

PARTS USED Flowering tops.

ACTIONS Antidepressant, anti-inflammatory, antiviral, analgesic, vulnerary, nerve tonic.

INDICATIONS Nerve pain, sciatica, neuralgia, shingles, depression, anxiety, wounds, burns, PMS, viral infections, cold sores, menopausal symptoms.

DESCRIPTION St John's wort grows up to 3 feet high and has opposite, stalkless leaves that are ½ to ¾ inch long. The leaves are dotted with tiny oil glands that look like perforations, giving it the botanical name *perforatum*. The flowers have five bright yellow petals that bear tiny black dots along the edge. There are many similar-looking plants of the *Hypericum* genus, but a distinguishing factor of *H. perforatum* is the presence of the oil glands and two opposite ridges that can be felt running up the stem. Some of the closely related species can also be used, so long as the flowering tips turn red when crushed. Harvest the flowering tips just as they flower in midsummer.

USES St. John's wort has long been prized as a wound herb. Today it is most famous for its antidepressant effects and there has been lots of research around the mood-enhancing effects of this unassuming herb. Studies have shown that extracts of St. John's wort are superior to a placebo in the treatment of mild to moderate depression. It has also been found to be similar in effect to some standard prescription antidepressant drugs but with fewer side effects. St. John's wort's use is not limited to depression for mood disorders; it is of benefit in nervousness, anxiety, and seasonal affective disorder (SAD). If sunshine could be bottled, it would come in the form of St. John's wort tincture.

Traditionally, St. John's wort was deemed at its most medicinally potent around the midsummer solstice, which falls between June 20th and June 22nd each year. It was held in such high esteem as a medicinal plant that, with the advent of Christianity, it became dedicated to St. John the Baptist, whose saint day falls on June 24th.

St. John's wort contains rutin, a constituent that has a firming effect on the veins and capillaries, making it a useful remedy for strengthening varicose veins and toning the uterus where there is heavy bleeding or painful periods. In fact, it is highly beneficial for the female reproductive system as a whole, reducing symptoms of PMS, hormonal mood disruption, and menopausal anxiety.

For viral infections such as cold sores and shingles, take St. John's wort internally as a tea or tincture, and apply the infused oil or balm directly to lesions to bring down pain and inflammation.

The internal use of St John's wort can cause photosensitivity in some, making the skin more sensitive to sunburn. Paradoxically, the infused oil used externally is a great remedy for sunburn and does not seem to cause the same sensitivity to the sun.

It is unparalleled as a remedy for wound healing, especially post-surgery. It was once regarded as an herb for both emotional and physical trauma and was used on the battlefield for deep puncture wounds. It relieves nerve pain and inflammation and encourages healing. Traditionally, fresh St. John's wort is steeped in olive oil using the sun infusion method on page 24 to make a beautiful bright red-infused oil for external use.

DOSAGE

INFUSION 1 teaspoon per 1 cup of boiling water; 1–3 cups per day.
TINCTURE ¼ to 1 teaspoon, up to three times daily.
Infused oil or balm: apply externally as needed.

CAUTIONS Contraindicated with many other drugs; check with your healthcare professional before taking internally if you are on any medications. St. John's wort may cause sensitivity to the sun. Not to be used in severe depression. Do not use during pregnancy, breastfeeding or for children without medical supervision.

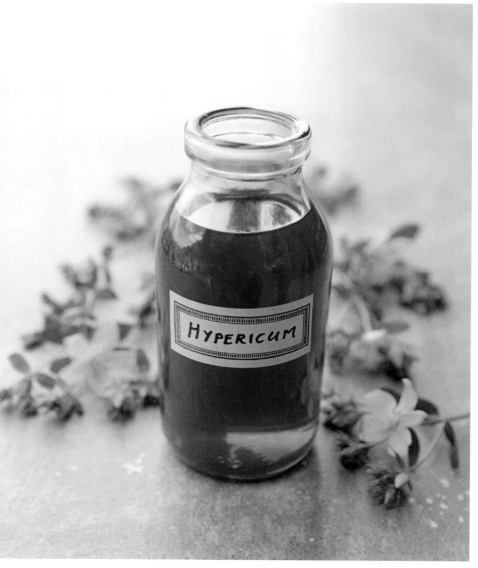

Inula helenium
Asteraceae

COMMON NAME Elecampane

PARTS USED Roots.

ACTIONS Expectorant, mucilaginous, astringent, antibacterial, digestive, antitussive, antiviral.

INDICATIONS Coughs, chest infections.

DESCRIPTION Elecampane is a large perennial plant growing up to 4 ½ feet tall, with flowers that look a little like a slimmer-petalled sunflower. The leaves are long, oval, and broad and can grow up to 12 inches in length.

USES Elecampane is a remedy for hard-to-shift and chronic lung conditions, including phlegmy coughs, chest infections, and asthma. It was previously even used to help treat tuberculosis before the discovery of antibiotics. You can feel its effect on the lungs by nibbling on a bit of root; the aroma clears the airways like a cough drop. The root is bitter as well as aromatic, and is especially helpful when appetite stimulation is needed; for example, after a cold or flu when lingering cough or phlegm inhibits a desire for food.

Traditionally, it was used to treat elf-shot, certain illnesses that were thought to be caused by being pierced with invisible arrows. Some herbalists think this may be a description of exhaustion or sapped energy, and explains the popular modern use for chronic fatigue and weakness.

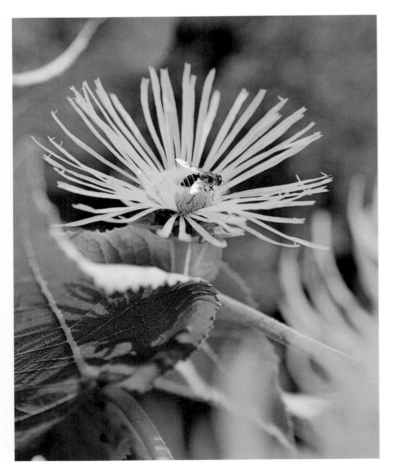

Juniperus communis
Cupressaceae

COMMON NAME Juniper

PARTS USED Fruit.

ACTIONS Urinary antiseptic, diuretic, carminative, antirheumatic, analgesic.

INDICATIONS Digestive upsets, urinary infections, muscle and period pain.

DESCRIPTION Juniper is a small coniferous shrub with needle-like leaves growing in whorls of three with a lighter central stripe. The highly aromatic fruits are found on the female plant and though initially green, ripen over a period of 1½ years. The fruits appear to be waxy purple berries but are actually small fleshy looking cones.

USES Juniper berries are commonly used in cooking due to their aromatic and spicy, warming volatile oils. These oils aid digestion through carminative and antiseptic actions, ideal for easing wind, colicky pains, and mild food poisoning. As an antiseptic, juniper can also be used for treating bacterial urinary tract infections.

Use an infused oil of juniper berry to make a comforting, circulatory rub, ideal for applying externally to painful muscles, joints, and period pain. Rub onto the area to warm and ease discomfort.

CAUTIONS Do not use in pregnancy or for those with kidney problems. Do not take for more than 6 weeks.

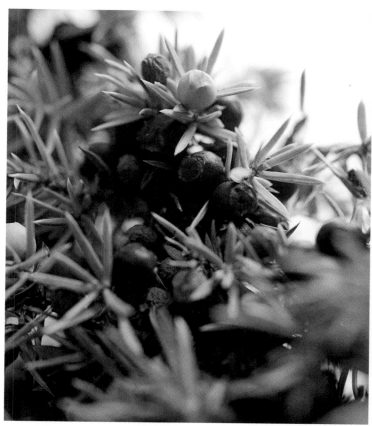

Lactuca virosa
Asteraceae

COMMON NAME Wild Lettuce

PARTS USED Leaves.

ACTIONS Sedative, analgesic, antispasmodic.

INDICATIONS Insomnia, pain relief, tense muscles.

DESCRIPTION This biennial plant belongs to the daisy family and grows tall and straight. It has many small, yellow, dandelion-like flowers and the seeds are similarly wind distributed via little fluffy parachutes. The long oval upper leaves have a row of soft spikes along the midrib and align themselves to follow the sun's pathway in a north-south direction, giving it its other name, compass plant.

USES Readers of Beatrix Potter's *The Tale of Peter Rabbit* will know that eating too much lettuce caused the Flopsy Bunnies to fall asleep! This is the main use of lettuce: it acts as a sedative and is useful when added to herbal infusions and tinctures for insomnia.

Wild lettuce is also a mild analgesic and antispasmodic; it relieves painful coughs, period pain, digestive discomfort, and tense muscles.

CAUTIONS Do not use in pregnancy or during lactation.

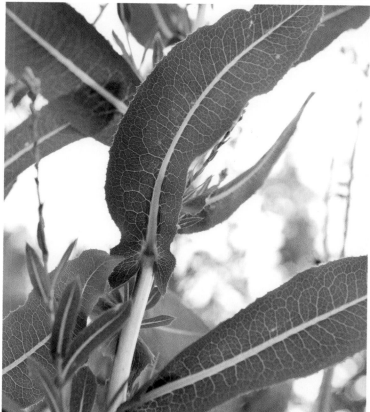

Lavandula angustifolia
Lamiaceae

COMMON NAME Lavender

PARTS USED Flowers.

ACTIONS Nervine, analgesic, antispasmodic, digestive, carminative, sedative, antidepressant, diaphoretic, expectorant, antimicrobial.

INDICATIONS Insomnia, stress, anxiety, headaches, digestive upsets, skin-calming.

DESCRIPTION Lavender is a shrubby, perennial herb indigenous to the Mediterranean but found all over the world as a popular garden plant. The leaves are small, lanceolate, and silvery green. The flowers are borne on long stems that pop up above the foliage, with a spike-like whorl of blue-purple flowers. The entire plant is aromatic.

USES One of the most popular uses of lavender throughout history has been as a fragrance herb for clothes, rooms, and toiletries. Its fresh floral scent is soothing and calming and is one of the first remedies turned to for aiding sleep and relaxation. It is commonly available as an essential oil for oil burners, inhalations, and external remedies, but the plant itself should not be overlooked. The flowers can be used in infusions and tinctures to improve sleep quality and ease stress-induced pressure headaches, tense muscles, and palpitations due to anxiety. For a tranquil nighttime drink, try the Chamomile Bedtime Latte (see page 127) and add ½ teaspoon of lavender flowers too!

The calming effect of lavender can also be used in respiratory disorders. Use the oil in inhalations and oil burners to encourage deep, relaxed breathing. It can be infused in oil and added to balms to soothe chest muscles tired from coughing. As an infusion or tincture, its antimicrobial, diaphoretic, decongestant, and expectorant actions are beneficial for cough remedies. The antibacterial properties mean it can also be used in cases of mild diarrhea and nausea, and will relieve pain and colicky symptoms.

Lavender can be added to face washes and creams to cool inflamed skin conditions, calming acne, eczema, and rosacea. The essential oil is also vital in a first aid cabinet; it can be diluted in a carrier oil and applied to burns to help reduce pain and scarring.

LAVENDER AROMATIC WATER

The soothing, calming, and cooling properties of lavender can be used in an aromatic water. Traditionally made using a still, you can make your own at home using everyday kitchen equipment, following one of these three quick and easy alternative methods.

Use the aromatic water to bathe inflamed skin, or add it to a spray bottle to mist on faces and pillows to ease stress and promote relaxation. You can make floral water with any aromatic herbs. Try rose petals or rosemary to help with memory.

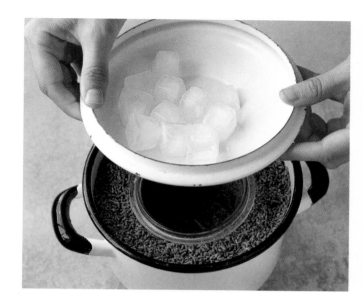

1 tablespoon vodka (or other clear alcohol)
10 drops of lavender essential oil
½ cup filtered water

Pour the vodka into a sterilized glass spray bottle and add the lavender essential oil (the clear alcohol allows the oil to disperse through the water). Top up with the filtered water, shaking to mix. Seal, label and date.

Keep in the fridge. Use the aromatic water as needed.

SHELF LIFE Up to 1 month in the fridge.

METHOD 2

½ cup filtered water
3 tablespoons fresh or dried lavender flowers

Pour the filtered water into a small pan and bring to a boil. Place the lavender flowers in a heatproof glass bowl, then carefully pour the boiling water over them. Cover with a plate to allow any condensation to drip back down into the bowl, then leave to cool or leave overnight.

Strain and discard the herb. Transfer the aromatic water into a sterilized glass spray bottle, seal, label and date.

Keep in the fridge. Use as needed.

SHELF LIFE Up to 1 week in the fridge.

METHOD 3

This method is the closest to distilling and uses everyday kitchen equipment. You'll need a saucepan with a lid that you can invert, ideally a dome-shaped lid, and a heatproof glass bowl that is small enough to fit inside this saucepan, leaving some space around the sides.

1 ¼ cups filtered water (plus extra for topping up)
a few big handfuls of fresh or dried lavender flowers
plenty of ice cubes

Pour the filtered water into the saucepan. Place the glass bowl in the center of the pan, then place the lavender flowers around the outside of the bowl, so that they cover the water but don't fill the pan. Put the lid, upside-down, onto the saucepan, then fill the inverted lid with ice cubes.

Gently heat the pan to a low simmer and then allow the steam to condense for 30 minutes. The evaporating water, with all the properties of the lavender, will hit the upside down pan lid and condense because the lid is iced. The condensed water will run down the lid and drip into the glass bowl.

Keep an eye on the water level throughout, topping it up if necessary, taking care not to lose too much precious steam as you do so. As the ice melts, periodically top up the lid with more ice, pouring away the melted ice before you add more.

Leonurus cardiaca
Lamiaceae

COMMON NAME Motherwort

PARTS USED Leaves and flowers.

ACTIONS Anti-anxiety, cardiac tonic, menstrual tonic, nervine.

INDICATIONS Menstrual problems, menopausal symptoms, anxiety, palpitations, blood pressure.

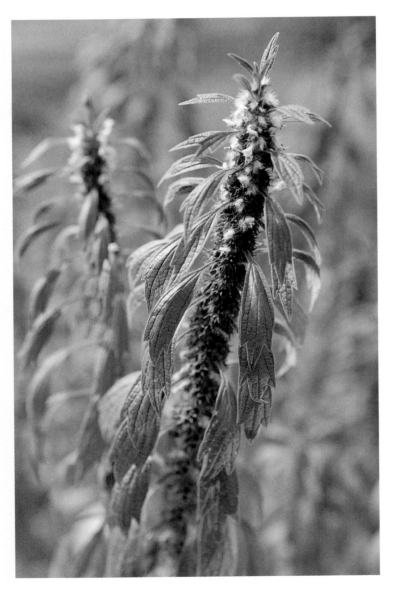

DESCRIPTION Motherwort is a member of the mint family with square stems and opposite leaves. The leaves are slim, palmate and have three lobes near to the top of the plant but produce more lobes going down toward the base; nearer the bottom, they look like a motherly hand held out ready to help! The flowers grow in whorls around the stem and are a distinctive two-lipped shape with appealing pink fluffy petals.

USES The name *motherwort* means "herb for mothers" and is used for menstrual problems and during labor. Culpeper says "it makes women joyful mothers of children" due to its nervine and hormone-balancing properties. It is an excellent menstrual tonic and encourages proper flow, so is used for women who have light but painful periods. It is also a useful remedy for PMS and for easing tension and anxiety during menopause.

The Latin name *cardiaca* refers to its use as a heart tonic. It is used for mild heart disorders, high and low blood pressure, and palpitations associated with thyroid conditions and anxiety.

CAUTION Because it is a uterine stimulant, it should be avoided in pregnancy.

Lonicera periclymenum,
L. caprifolium, L. japonica
Caprifoliaceae

COMMON NAMES Honeysuckle, Woodbine

PARTS USED Flowers, leaves.

ACTIONS Cooling, antiseptic, anti-asthmatic, analgesic, antispasmodic.

INDICATIONS Coughs, mouth ulcers, gum disease, sore throats, fever, hot flashes, urinary tract infections.

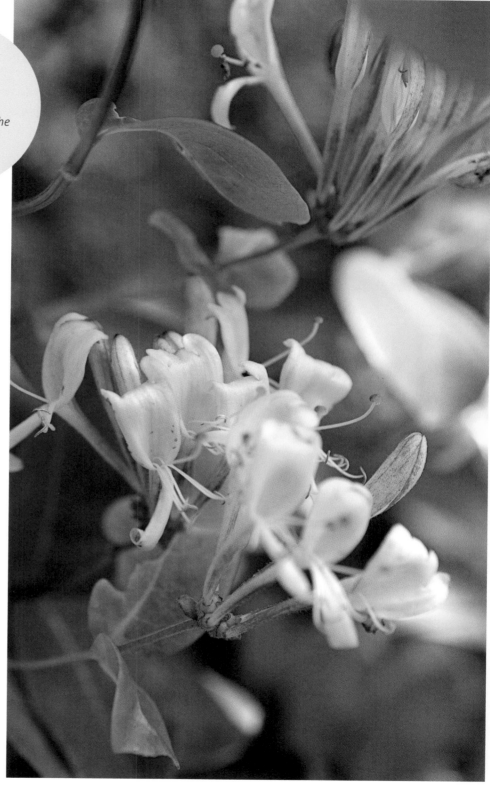

TIP
Try honeysuckle-infused honey for sore throats using the recipe on page 19.

DESCRIPTION A common garden climbing plant. The leaves are oval and opposite. The clusters of fragrant, trumpet-shaped flowers range in color from cream to deep yellow/pink, with red and purple garden varieties. The yellow-pink varieties can be used medicinally. Fruits form as poisonous orange-red berries.

USES The flowers and leaves of honeysuckle contain salicylic acid, a compound in aspirin that helps bring down inflammation and reduce pain. It has been prized throughout history as a deeply cooling plant and was employed to treat menopausal hot flashes, fever, and other heated conditions.

The flowers of honeysuckle have a long history of use in asthmatic and respiratory conditions. A honey or syrup made from the flowers is antiseptic and reduces spasm, helping to soothe a dry, irritated cough and sore throat. The leaves of honeysuckle are astringent and antiseptic; these can be decocted and made into a gargle to soothe inflamed tissues in sore throats, mouth ulcers, and gum disease.

Matricaria chamomilla;
Chamaemelum nobile
Asteraceae

COMMON NAMES German Chamomile; Roman Chamomile

PARTS USED Flowers.

ACTIONS Antimicrobial, anti-inflammatory, antispasmodic, anxiolytic, digestive.

INDICATIONS Indigestion, digestive upsets, anxiety, stress, insomnia, skin irritation, wound healing.

DESCRIPTION Chamomile flowers have a daisy-like yellow button center surrounded with white petals. When crushed, they usually have a sweet apple-like scent. Other chamomiles include Pineappleweed (*Matricaria discoidea*) and other scentless varieties. Any scented versions can be used interchangeably with the German and Roman varieties, though they have a milder effect.

USES German and Roman (pictured right) are the two main medicinally used chamomiles and are good all-round, safe herbs that are essential for the herbal medicine cabinet.

Chamomile has a long history of medicinal use with evidence of use in archaeological sites dating back to Neanderthal times. It is a palatable herb with a fruity, mildly bitter flavor and anti-inflammatory actions that make it a fabulous medicine for a wide range of disorders, from skin problems to anxiety and digestive upsets.

The aromatic essential oils are antimicrobial and relaxant, so are particularly useful for disorders of the digestive system. A strong infusion will ease indigestion, griping pain, nausea, and diarrhea.

The relaxing and soothing properties of chamomile make it an excellent calming remedy for stressed or upset people, and it's particularly safe for children. Because it also aids sleep, a hot chamomile water or milk infusion before bed is good for insomnia and is useful for fretful, feverish children in cases of colds and flu.

Chamomile is one of the top skin herbs in an herbalist's repertoire for both beauty and medicine. It is anti-inflammatory and calming for inflamed skin, infected cuts, and chronic skin problems. The essential oil of German chamomile contains constituents called chamazulene and azulene, which turn a deep blue color during the distillation process. This beautiful oil has excellent healing properties; add it to creams that call for a powerful anti-inflammatory action for conditions such as acne, rosacea, eczema, and psoriasis. The flowers can also be used simply and effectively in an infusion to make a wash or steam for the same conditions.

Chamomile infusion has a traditional use for colicky or teething babies; a mild infusion can be taken in milk, or a clean flannel soaked in the infusion and frozen makes a soothing and calming chew.

CAUTION Some people are allergic to the *Asteraceae* daisy family and it should be avoided in these cases.

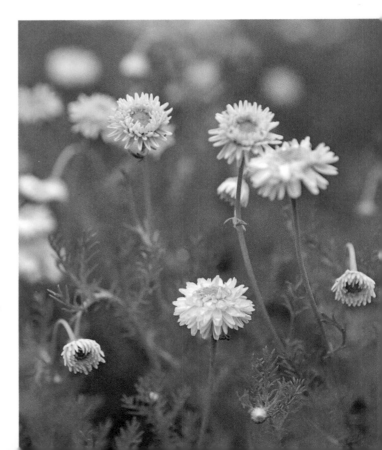

CHAMOMILE BEDTIME LATTE

This calming milky drink is served warm and is ideal as a comforting, bedtime soother.

1 ½ cups cow's or goat's milk (or use a non-dairy alternative, such as almond or soy milk)
1 teaspoon dried or 2 teaspoons fresh chamomile flowers
honey, to taste

Place the milk and chamomile flowers in a small pan, bring slowly to a simmer, then simmer gently for 5 minutes.

Strain into a mug, stir in honey to taste, and enjoy the drink an hour before going to bed.

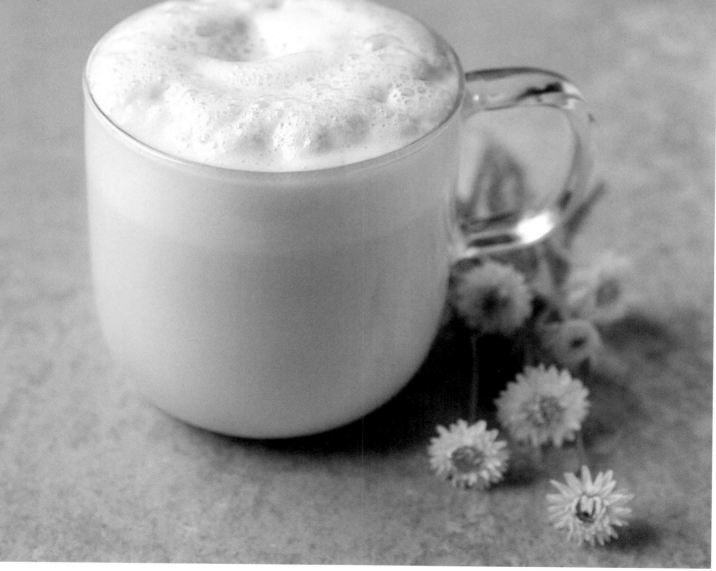

Melissa officinalis
Lamiaceae

COMMON NAMES Lemon Balm, Bee Balm

PARTS USED Leaves.

ACTIONS Nervine, carminative, mood-lifting, diaphoretic, hypotensive, antiviral.

INDICATIONS Cold sores, anxiety, panic attacks, low mood, high blood pressure, colds, flu, shingles.

DESCRIPTION A bushy perennial of the mint family, reaching a height of up to 3 feet. Leaves are bright green, opposite, toothed and lemon-scented. The stems are square. Lemon balm's two-lipped flowers are white and grow in whorls from the leaf axis.

USES The Latin name *Melissa* derives from the Greek *mel* meaning honey or bee. When crushed or rubbed between the fingers, the leaves of lemon balm release a delightful, floral-lemony scent that bees and humans alike are drawn to.

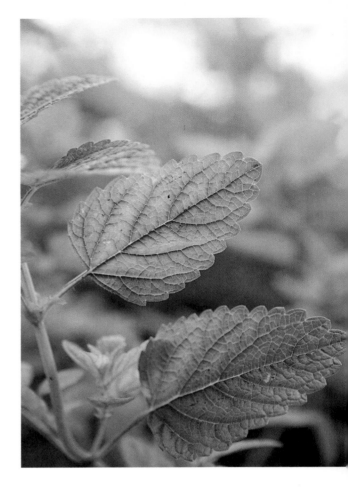

The heavenly smell of lemon balm comes from its content of volatile oils, which are responsible for many of its medicinal properties. These oils dissipate particularly quickly when lemon balm is dried and so it is best to use it fresh where possible. It can be made into syrups, tinctures, or honey, or frozen in ice cube trays to preserve its fresh lemon scent.

Being an aromatic plant, it acts as a carminative, relieving spasms in the digestive tract and dispersing wind. It is especially helpful for digestive problems that are exacerbated by stress or mood.

The calming effects of lemon balm extend to the nervous system, where it is used for anxiety and panic attacks, particularly where there is rapid heartbeat or palpitations. It may be added to herbal tea or tincture mixes for high blood pressure associated with stress. One of its more traditional uses was as a longevity herb. Paracelsus, a sixteenth-century physician, believed it would "revivify" the tired and strengthen the brain. It is a great herb to use in exam stress or when a work deadline looms, as it aids concentration and soothes the mind without being overly sedating.

Lemon balm's volatile oils are also highly antiviral and it can be used internally and externally. The infused oil can be applied to viral skin conditions such as shingles. A lip balm made from the infused oil (see recipe opposite) can help to prevent and lessen the duration of cold sores. Its antiviral effects, coupled with mild diaphoretic action, can help to bring down fever and infection in colds and flu.

MELISSA LIP BALM

This lip balm contains moisturizing oils and antiviral St. John's wort, lemon balm and eucalyptus. Eucalyptus may not be the first scent you think of when deciding on a lip balm flavor, but it is full of antiviral agents that blitz the cold sore virus. It also gives the lips a fresh and tingly feeling.

2 ounces shea butter
¼ ounce beeswax
2 teaspoons lemon balm-infused oil
10 drops of St John's wort tincture
10 drops of eucalyptus essential oil

Melt the shea butter, beeswax and lemon balm-infused oil together in a bain-marie.

Remove from the heat and whisk in the St. John's wort tincture and eucalyptus essential oil.

Pour into small pots or lip balm tubes, seal, label and date.

To use, apply throughout the day, as and when needed, as you would any lip balm.

SHELF LIFE Up to 1 year (store as you would any lip balm).

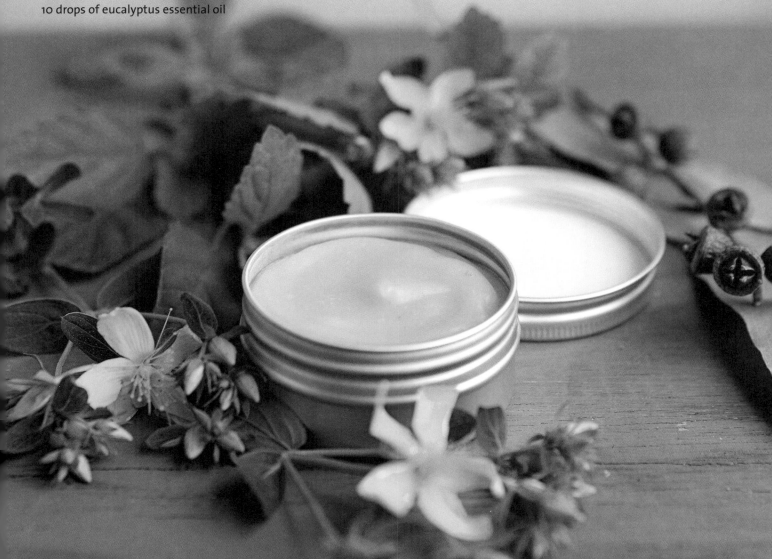

Plantago spp.
(P. lanceolata, P. major, P. media)
Plantaginaceae

COMMON NAMES Plantain: Ribwort, Broadleaf, and Hoary

PARTS USED Leaves: dry them quickly otherwise they discolor.

ACTIONS Expectorant, demulcent, astringent, vulnerary, diuretic, alterative, antiviral.

INDICATIONS Cuts, wounds, insect bites, sinusitis, hay fever, coughs, chest infections, urinary infections, digestive upsets.

DESCRIPTION Plantain is a biennial meadow flower that likes to grow along well-trodden pathways across fields and gardens. This is because it has a sticky seed that spreads by hitching a lift on the soles of shoes. All the species have a dense green leaf that grows in a basal rosette and has thick ribs running parallel along the blade. These veins are particularly noticeable along the back of the leaf and are a useful identifying feature.

The leaf of the ribwort (*P. lanceolata*) has long thin leaves; the broadleaf species (*P. major*) are roundish or spade-like and stemmed. The flowers of the two differ slightly; the ribwort has a tall stem ending in a roundish spike of tiny greenish-brown flowers that produce a "corona" or Saturn-ring of stamens. The broadleaf plantain, on the other hand, has a longer, thin green spike of flowers that look like one of its folk names: "rats-tails".

The hoary plantain (*P. media*) has leaves and flowers that are in between the two other species. The leaves are broad and long, and the flowers have a brush-like corona of purplish stamens. However, all these species of plantain can be used interchangeably.

USES Plantain was recorded as a sacred herb in Anglo-Saxon times and is still a top first aid plant for herbalists today, with a wide range of applications. It has both demulcent and astringent properties, which give it a soothing yet toning action on inflamed membranes.

It can be simply used fresh on insect bites and cuts for itching and wound healing; crush a clean leaf well to extract the juice and apply to the area. Its wound-healing abilities may be attributed to aucubin, an antimicrobial constituent, and allantoin, also found in comfrey, which encourages tissue repair and modulates inflammation. Its ability to heal inflamed tissues including mucous membranes, combined with anti-allergic properties, means it is a great remedy for ear infections, sinusitis, and hay fever. Use the tincture internally for ear infections or combine in an infusion with elderflower and nettle for a traditional hay fever remedy.

Plantain leaf infusion can be used for urinary tract infections, and has an expectorant action for coughs and chest infections. Its anti-inflammatory healing means it can also be taken for soothing upset digestion after vomiting and diarrhea.

Plantain may appear to be a plain weed and a nuisance in some lawns, but it is a valuable medicine and deserves a place in the home remedy cabinet.

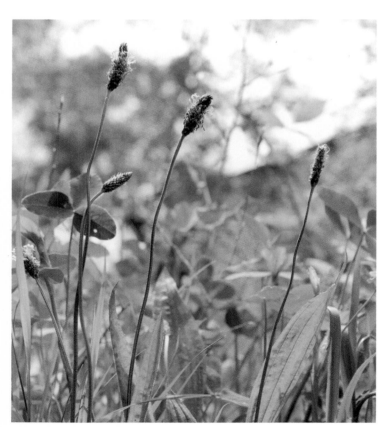

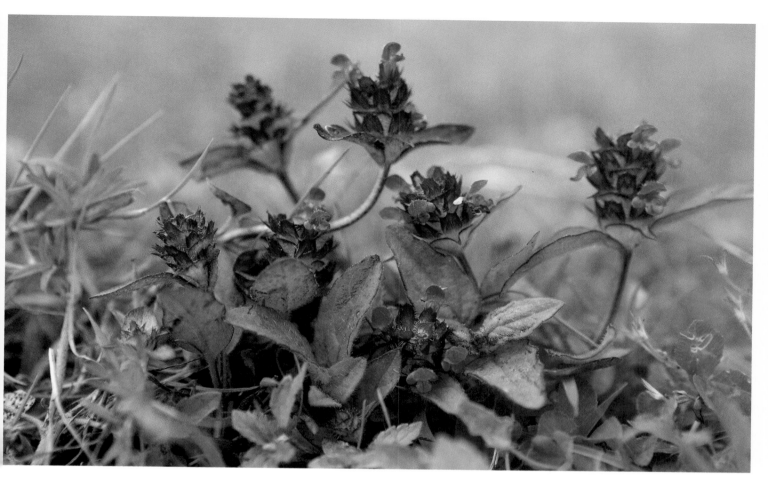

Prunella vulgaris
Lamiaceae

COMMON NAME Self-heal

PARTS USED Leaves and flowers.

ACTIONS Styptic, antimicrobial, bitter, diuretic, hypotensive.

INDICATIONS Cuts and wounds, hemorrhoids, high blood pressure, heavy menstruation, colds, flu, mouth ulcers, hot flashes.

DESCRIPTION A small perennial herb of grasslands and fields with creeping roots and square stems. The plant is small and stubby looking with small, opposite, and lanceolate leaves. The top two leaves grow like a collar directly under a spike-like, squareish whorl of flowers. The flowers are asymmetrical with two-lobed blue-purple petals.

USES The common name of this plant recalls its once well known use as a cure-all. It is an excellent wound healer, styptic, and antiseptic, and was known as "carpenter's herb" for its effects on healing deep, sharp cuts. It can be crushed and applied fresh as a poultice on wounds, grazes, bruises, boils and mouth ulcers. Use in lotions and creams for all-year-round healing and for treating hemorrhoids. As a styptic, it reduces bleeding and helps to reduce heavy menstruation.

Make an infusion with hawthorn and linden blossom to lower high blood pressure, cool hot flashes, and soothe irritability, anxiety and overexcitability, particularly in children. Self-heal is also used for viral infections from colds, flu, and cold sores and helps to ease sore and swollen throats.

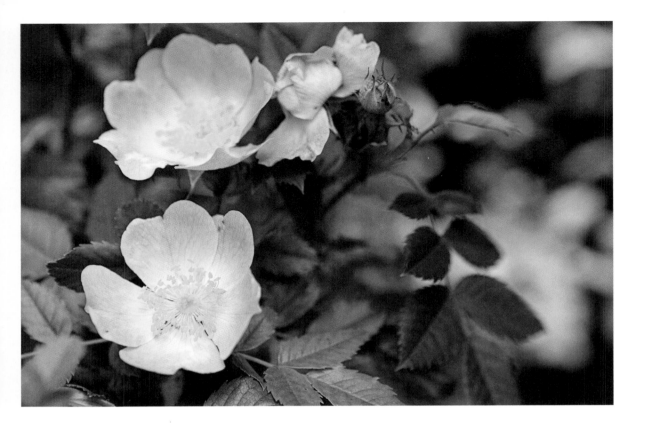

Rosa spp.
(R. damascena, R. gallica, R. canina)
Rosaceae

COMMON NAMES Rose, Damascus Rose, Wild Rose, Dog Rose

PARTS USED Flowers, top leaves, hips.

ACTIONS Astringent, anti-inflammatory, diuretic, sedative, anxiolytic.

INDICATIONS Anxiety, grief, PMS, menopausal anxiety, colds, flu, sore throats, diarrhea, skin and joint health, arthritis.

DESCRIPTION Roses have five-petaled flowers with multiple stamens that give the center a bushy look. The petals are usually white or pink and often beautifully scented. Cultivated roses have numerous petals because of the way they have been bred for show, but as long as they are scented (and have not been sprayed with pesticides), they can still be used. The leaves are compound with 5–7 leaflets. The long tough stems clamber over hedges and walls using their large, hooked thorns. The fruit is a "hip" that looks like a round or oval capsule and turns red once ripe. The hips contain little seeds with irritating hairs that were once used in itching powder; these need to be processed out before use.

There are many wild varieties including the common dog rose (*R. canina*) and sweet briar (*R. rubiginosa*); these are the two most used medicinally for their hips. *R. damascena* and *R. gallica* are traditionally cultivated medicinal roses famous for their heavenly scented, numerous petals.

USES What summer in a country garden would be complete without scented roses? Even Shakespeare described Titania's fairy bower scene with the beautiful and evocative rose, and it has long been associated with love and beauty. It is the sweet and distinctive scent that has helped establish rose as a popular medicine and beauty product around the world for thousands of years. Scented aromatic waters are a popular way to take roses, but tinctures and infusions are also effective. They are used for calming and uplifting anxious minds, for the female reproductive system, and to comfort those stricken with grief.

The flowers and upper leaves are used as a mild astringent for tightening tissues and inflamed skin problems, sore throats, digestive upsets and mild diarrhea. Try a rosebud infusion or create a delicious elixir with the most fragrant petals using brandy and honey, and use it for a medicinal pick-me-up in cases of shock or low feelings. Alternatively, dry the petals and then grind to a powder in a blender. Warm some honey until it is runny, then add your powdered rose petals to create a thick paste. Take a spoonful for sore throats, upset tummies, and when you feel down.

Rose has a hormonal-balancing effect on the female reproductive system, regulating periods and lessening premenstrual and menopausal irritability. It is particularly effective if used both internally in infusions or tinctures and externally as an uplifting aromatic spray.

The hips are high in nutrients and antioxidants and have been traditionally used to make a syrup for its high vitamin C content, as a laxative for constipation, and for helping reduce the symptoms of colds and flu. The rosehip syrup is particularly suitable for children as it is a safe and tasty remedy. The hips contain flavonoids, which are powerful anti-inflammatories, and when combined with the natural vitamin C content, aid collagen formation and help with painful joints and arthritic conditions.

The hips are best gathered after the first frost when the flesh has softened, making them sweeter, but they need to be processed to remove the irritant seed hairs. If you would like to use them before the first frost, place them in the freezer for a short time (to mimic a frost), but do not allow them to freeze solid.

ROSEHIP POWDER

This vitamin-rich powder is made with the whole rosehip, including the seeds, but the hairs are carefully removed. It can be sprinkled on food or put into capsules and is an excellent remedy for arthritic conditions.

Rosehips

Pick as many rosehips as you need, then rinse and dry them. Spread them out on a tray and leave in a warm place until dehydrated and hard. This may take up to around 1 week, depending on the ambient temperature. If the weather is damp, use a dehydrator or a very low oven to do this.

Once the hips are completely dry, pulse them in a blender until they are broken into largish pieces (this is to make sure the flesh will not pass through a strainer).

Carefully take the chopped pieces and place them in a strainer over a piece of newspaper, so you can sift out the irritating seed hairs from the rose hip seeds and skin. Discard the dust and hairs collected in the newspaper, being careful not to breathe in the irritating hairs.

Retain the rest of the material in the strainer, making sure no hairs remain, then re-blend this to a powder. Transfer the powder to a sterilized jar, then seal, label and date.

Use the rosehip powder to sprinkle over food (use it like salt and pepper on savory food or sprinkle over desserts) or put it into infusions.

SHELF LIFE Up to 1 year in a cool, dark place.

Alternatively, combine the rosehip powder with enough honey to make a stiff paste and then roll into small, pea-size balls to make pills (like in the Slippery Elm, Meadowsweet, and Milk Thistle Soothing Lozenges – see page 143). Leave these to dry fully and then keep in an airtight container in the fridge for up to 6 months.

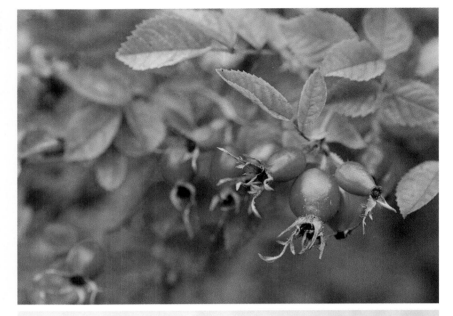

HIP AND HAW KETCHUP

Pick the rosehips for this recipe after the first frost when the berries have softened and sweetened slightly. This delicious rosehip and hawthorn ketchup combines the nutrient-rich wild berries of autumn with warming herbs and spices. Use it as you would tomato ketchup, and it also makes a great accompaniment to cheeses.

10 ounces rosehips
7 ounces hawthorns
½ cup water
1 ¼ cups apple cider vinegar
1 medium onion, diced
2 garlic cloves, crushed
1 teaspoon allspice powder
½ teaspoon cayenne pepper
1 teaspoon sea salt
⅔ cup dark brown sugar

Place all the ingredients except the brown sugar in a pan, cover with a tight-fitting lid, bring to a boil and simmer gently for 15–20 minutes, until the fruits have softened.

Pour the mixture into a strainer, set over a bowl and rub the flesh of the fruit through with a wooden spoon, discarding the pips and skins. Line another strainer with cheesecloth, set over a pan, and pass the pulp through once again to remove any rosehip hairs. Add the sugar to the pan and simmer gently for an additional 5–10 minutes, stirring constantly. Pour the hot mixture into sterilized jars or bottles, seal and allow to cool.

SHELF LIFE Store in the fridge unopened for up to 1 year. Once opened, use within 1 month.

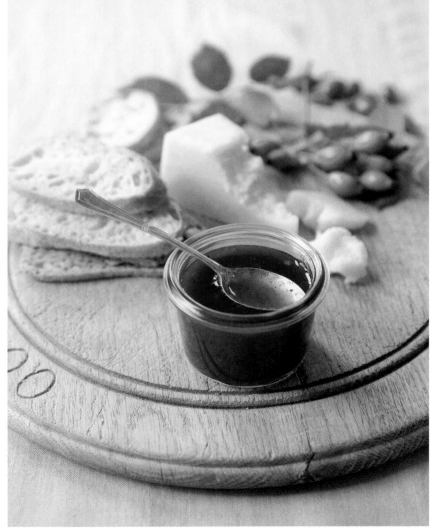

Rubus fruticosus
Rosaceae

COMMON NAMES Blackberry, Bramble

PARTS USED Flowers, leaves, young shoots, berries.

ACTIONS Astringent, nutritive, vulnerary, styptic.

INDICATIONS Diarrhea, sore throats, gum disease, sunburn, cuts and scrapes, heavy periods.

DESCRIPTION A perennial, sprawling bush, with thick purplish green stems covered with sharp thorns. The white or light pink, five-petaled flowers of spring later bear juicy, purple black berries. Brambles hybridize prolifically, making the leaf shape and form extremely variable. Mostly the leaves are compound, dark green, sometimes with a red hue, and have five leaflets in the first year's growth and three on the second year's fruiting branches.

USES Brambles are a highly successful species that can be found in most temperate regions of the globe, loved by some and loathed by others. They provide an ample supply of food and medicine but are also highly invasive, particularly to newly cleared land, much to the gardener's dismay. However, in the wild, they perform an important ecological role, protecting young tree saplings from grazing animals to allow new forest growth.

Brambles give us medicine throughout most of the year. In the spring, we use the shoots and baby leaves, which are cleansing, nutritive, and gently astringent. In the summer, the older, more powerfully astringent leaves can also be harvested. In the late summer, the berries are abundant and full of antioxidants and vitamin C.

The leaves of brambles are high in tannins that tighten and soothe inflamed tissues. Combine them with other antimicrobial herbs, like thyme or sage, in a gargle for sore throats and bleeding gums.

Crushed blackberry leaves placed over cuts and wounds act as a styptic to stop bleeding and promote scab formation; the perfect remedy for scratches acquired during blackberry picking! The cooled infusion can be soaked in cotton and swabbed over sunburn to relieve soreness and calm redness. Young blackberry leaves can be used in a similar way to raspberry leaf in toning the uterus and relieving heavy periods.

Bramble is surrounded by much folklore and was once considered a sacred herb by many cultures. It was said that blackberries must not be picked or eaten after Michaelmas, the feast of Saint Michael on 29th September, because "the devil spits on them". This superstition makes sense because in many countries, the first frosts start around then, after which time the berries ferment and go moldy.

When picking blackberries, they should come off the plant quite easily; if you have to pull hard or snap them off, they are likely to be unripe. Check the heel (the place where the berries connect to the plant). It should be pale green or white; if dark or brown, they are overripe and no good for use.

It is not just the berries that are edible on brambles; the inner flesh of the spring stems is crisp and tasty eaten raw, lightly steamed or added to stir-fries. As are the very young leaf shoots. Just be sure to remove any thorns first!

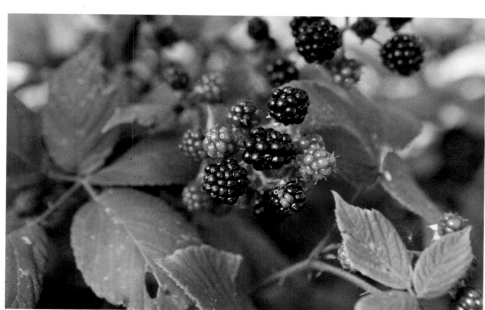

BLACKBERRY AND RASPBERRY OXYMEL

Oxymels are a mixture of honey and vinegar that make a traditional, delicious summer drink popular with the ancient Romans. Add to salad dressings or use as a refreshing cordial mixed with sparkling water. Blackberries and raspberries are high in vitamins and minerals. They are also astringent, and the vinegar and honey in this recipe add their own cooling, healing properties. Use diluted as a gargle for sore throats or in a hot drink for reducing fever in colds and flu.

8 ounces fresh blackberries
8 ounces fresh raspberries
organic apple cider vinegar, to cover
honey

Fill a sterilized Mason jar loosely with the fruit, then cover with vinegar. Seal and leave to infuse for 1 month, gently turning periodically.

After a month, strain the mixture, reserving the infused vinegar and discarding the fruit.

Mix equal parts of the vinegar and honey together, then pour into a sterilized bottle. Seal, label and date.

To use, take 2 teaspoons diluted in a little cold water or add 2 teaspoons to an infusion, 1–3 times daily.

SHELF LIFE Keep (unopened) in a cool, dark place for up to 6 months. Once opened, keep in the fridge and use within 3 months.

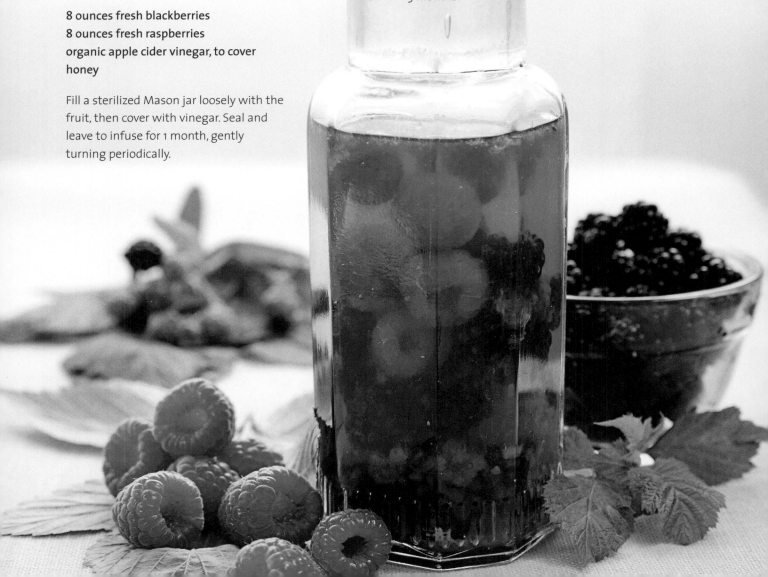

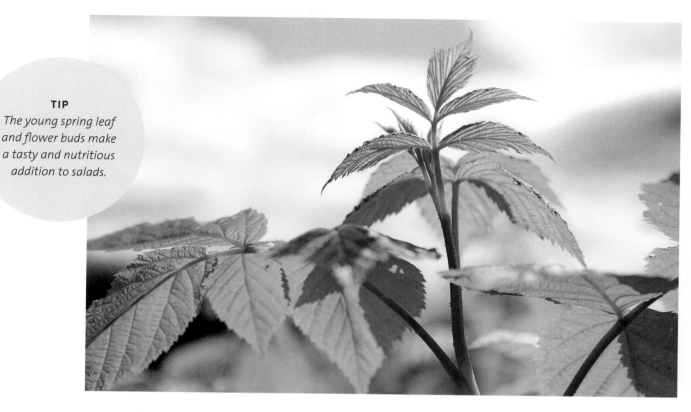

TIP
The young spring leaf and flower buds make a tasty and nutritious addition to salads.

Rubus idaeus
Rosaceae

COMMON NAME Raspberry

PARTS USED Young leaves, berries.

ACTIONS Astringent, tonic, antispasmodic, uterine tonic.

INDICATIONS Heavy periods, painful periods, childbirth, post-labor, sore throats, mouth ulcers, gum disease, diarrhea.

DESCRIPTION A thorny shrub similar in appearance to the bramble but more delicate-looking and with less menacing thorns. Leaves are palmate and light green with silvery undersides. The symmetrical flowers have five white or pink-tinged petals with numerous stamens that later become sweet, fleshy red fruits.

USES Raspberry leaf is gentle, toning, and nutritive. It has high concentrations of calcium and other minerals, making it a good all-round tonic. An infusion of the leaves can be taken to strengthen the muscles of the uterus, reducing pain and heavy bleeding during menstruation. Traditionally, it was taken during the last trimester of pregnancy to prepare the body for childbirth, toning the uterine and abdominal muscles and reducing the chances of hemorrhage, making for an easier delivery. Post-labor, it helps to firm up loose muscles and skin as well as promote breast milk production. It is the young leaves of the wild raspberry that are commonly used medicinally, but cultivated varieties are also effective.

Raspberry leaf tea makes an astringent and cooling gargle for sore throats, mouth ulcers, and gum disease. It is much gentler in its astringency than its cousin the bramble, and is a useful remedy for diarrhea in children and those with a delicate constitution.

The berries are delicious and high in antioxidants and vitamins, especially the wild varieties. They can be eaten straight from the bush, added to cakes, or made into an herbal vinegar in the same way as blackberries.

Rumex crispus
Polygonaceae

COMMON NAMES Curly Dock, Curled Dock

PARTS USED Roots.

ACTIONS Bitter, laxative, alterative, astringent.

INDICATIONS Appetite stimulant, digestive, constipation, boils, acne, eczema, psoriasis, arthritis.

DESCRIPTION Curly dock is a perennial plant with relatively large, shiny, oval, weathered-looking leaves arranged in a basal rosette. Curly dock leaves are distinguished from other docks by their wavy edges. The flowers are tiny, reddish green, and grow in spikes. The fruits are small, three-sided, and winged and look like a little person wearing a bonnet. Harvest the yellowest roots, as these will be the most bitter and medicinal.

USES Curly dock can often be found growing by nettles and is probably one of the most common plant remedies known— for the relief of nettle stings. However, it is the bitter-tasting root that is most used in herbal medicine. Its bitterness stimulates the liver and encourages the production of gastric juices to help improve digestion and absorption of nutrients. Through stimulating bile production, curly dock acts as a laxative. It contains some anthroquinone glycosides, which also have a laxative action but are slightly irritating to the digestive tract and should not be used continuously for constipation.

It has an alterative and cleansing effect on the blood and lymph systems, and combined with its laxative properties, helps rid the body of wastes. It is used by herbalists to treat chronic skin and joint problems including boils, acne, eczema, psoriasis and arthritis.

CAUTIONS Do not take during pregnancy or breastfeeding.

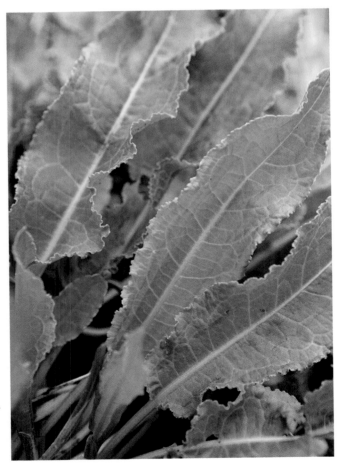

Scutellaria lateriflora
Lamiaceae

COMMON NAMES Skullcap, Mad Dog, Helmet Flower

PARTS USED Leaves and flowers.

ACTIONS Sedative, nerve tonic, adaptogen.

INDICATIONS Stress, fatigue, depression, anxiety, insomnia, muscle spasm, tremor, amenorrhea, PMS, teeth grinding.

DESCRIPTION A perennial herb growing to around $1\frac{1}{2}$ feet in height. Skullcap has opposite, pointed, toothed leaves. The hooded, two-lipped blue to purple flowers grow laterally along one side of the smooth, square stem, hence the plant's botanical name *lateriflora*.

USES Skullcap supports and nourishes the nervous system, helping the body to cope with physical and mental stress, particularly when it causes muscle spasm, headaches and teeth grinding. It has been used in nervous system conditions, such as multiple sclerosis, Tourette's syndrome, and Alzheimer's disease, to lessen muscle spasms and tremor. It is a slightly sedative herb and can be used long term to improve sleep quality and reduce hyperactivity and anxiety. An energetic use for skullcap is to relax and lessen overthinking, calming worried minds. This action is particularly useful when circulating thoughts before bedtime lead to insomnia.

While skullcap is noted for its sedative, relaxing effects, it also brings about focus. Studies have found that one of its constituents, scutellarin, improves blood flow to the brain, making it an excellent remedy for exam and work stress, when the nerves need calming, without being overly sedating.

Skullcap is the perfect remedy for hormonal stress and PMS. Traditionally, it was used by Native American peoples to regulate menstruation and relieve premenstrual tension.

Skullcap herb is best used fresh. Make a fresh tincture when the plant is in flower to preserve its medicinal qualities for year-round use.

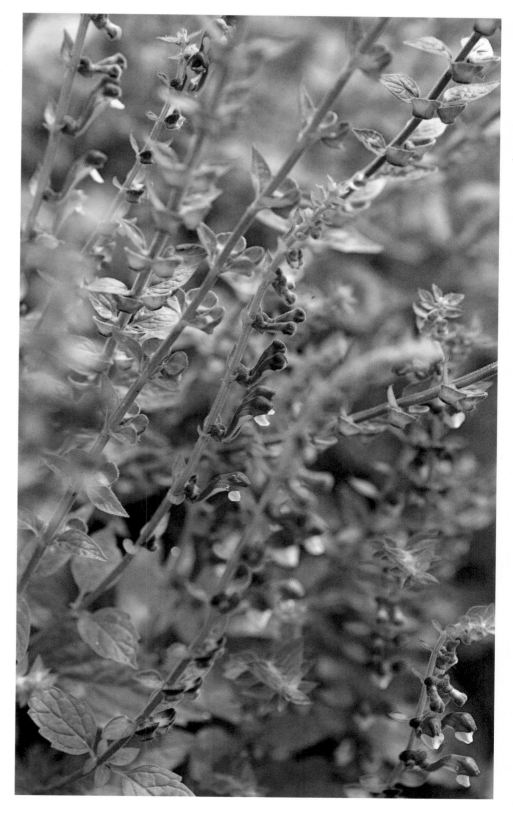

Silybum marianum
Asteracecae

COMMON NAME Milk Thistle

PARTS USED Leaves, seeds.

ACTIONS Bitter, hepatoprotectant, astringent, diuretic, milk stimulant.

INDICATIONS Hangovers, post-illness recovery, hormonal imbalance, skin disorders, breast milk production.

DESCRIPTION This plant belongs to the thistle tribe of the daisy family and has lots of familiar thistle features; prickly lobed leaves and an artichoke-style flower head surrounded by green bracts and capped with purple flowers that look like a fluffy beret. The seeds form on the flower head within the cup of the bracts, and range from pale to dark brown in a flask shape with a little pale "lid" at one end. One identifying feature that makes it different, however, is the markings on the leaves. The veins appear to be milky, or according to folklore, splashed with the "Virgin Mary's milk". This association with a deity highlights its importance in folk medicine.

USES A vital part of any herbalist's kit, milk thistle is a remedy specifically used for the liver. One of the constituents, silymarin, has been shown in scientific studies to help prevent liver cells from absorbing and being damaged by toxins caused by viruses and poisons. Another chemical, silybin, has been found to help protect against liver cirrhosis and mushroom poisoning. This supports its traditional use as a defense against and treatment of liver complaints. Practically, this means it is a good remedy to use for recuperation after illnesses, after some heavy medications (under supervision), and even for hangovers! It is bitter and so helps stimulate the liver and digestion to clear excess hormones and wastes from the body; it's also good for balancing the hormones and treating skin problems. The reference to the Virgin Mary's milk also echoes its other use for stimulating milk production in lactating mothers.

The seeds are the part used most medicinally, although if the thorns are removed from the leaves, the leaves can then be cooked lightly and eaten. A practical way to incorporate the seeds into a medicinal protocol is to put them into a pepper grinder to grind ½ teaspoon over each meal. For hangovers, protect your liver before a night out by chewing a spoonful of seeds, and take some more the next day: your liver will thank you for it!

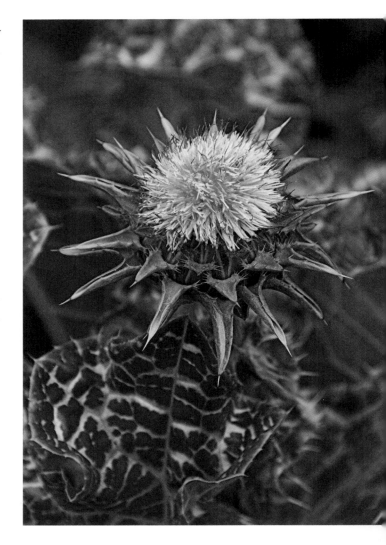

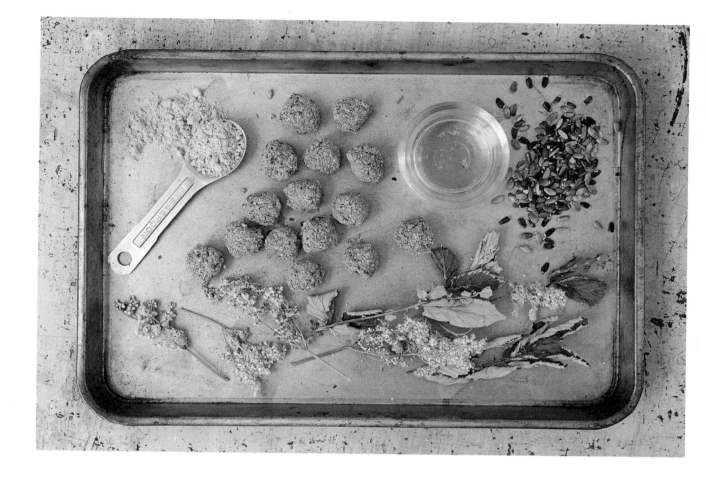

MEADOWSWEET AND MILK THISTLE SOOTHING LOZENGES

These are multipurpose, soothing lozenges that can be used for sore throats, coughs, heartburn, hyperacidity and vomiting (they work a charm for hangovers!).

⅓ ounce dried meadowsweet flowers (ensure all stems are removed)
⅓ ounce slippery elm or marshmallow root powder
⅓ ounce milk thistle powder
2 teaspoons honey

Place all the herbs in a small bowl. Mix the honey and 1 teaspoon of water together in a separate small bowl.

Slowly add enough of the honey mix to the herb mix, a little at a time, until a thick paste is formed.

Roll the paste into small, pea-size balls, place on a plate, and leave out (at room temperature) for a few days to dry. Store in an airtight container.

To use, suck, chew or swallow 2–3 lozenges with liquid per day, as needed.

SHELF LIFE Up to 6 months in a cool, dark place.

Stachys officinalis (syn. *Stachys betonica*)
Lamiaceae

COMMON NAME Wood Betony

PARTS USED Leaves and flowers.

ACTIONS Bitter, circulatory, nerve tonic.

INDICATIONS Headaches, anxiety and tension, insomnia, memory, bitter digestive.

DESCRIPTION A perennial meadow herb with square stems and oppositely arranged, slim, toothed leaves. The flowers are a brush-like spike of pinky-purplish, two-lipped flowers that grow up straight and tall.

USES In the past, wood betony was considered a powerful panacea and was added to protection amulets. Today, it is primarily used for insomnia and various types of headaches of different origins including anxiety, poor digestion, and migraines. Its essential oil content relaxes muscle tension and stimulates the circulation, while its bitter taste stimulates the digestive juices. To use, take a dropperful of the tincture in a little water as needed. For more intense headaches, combine it with a complementary herb, such as wild oats for nervous tension, or motherwort for hormonal headaches.

It is also beneficial for improving memory and can be used in infusions with other herbs, such as lemon balm, to make a relaxing tea ideal for students.

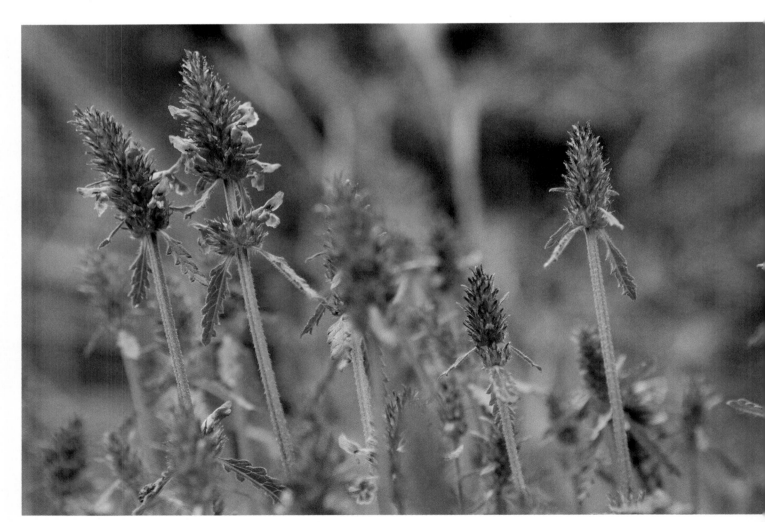

Stellaria media
Caryophyllaceae

COMMON NAMES Chickweed, Starweed

PARTS USED Whole fresh, aerial plant.

ACTIONS Anti-inflammatory, anti-itch, wound healing.

INDICATIONS Itchy rashes, eczema, psoriasis, chickenpox, abscesses, ulcers, burns, digestive irritation, convalescence.

DESCRIPTION This unassuming little plant loves growing in disturbed soil. Its numerous tiny white flowers give it its name *Stellaria media*, meaning "among the stars," though they usually open at midday! It has a single line of hairs that grows up the stem between each leaf node and swaps over to a different side after each leaf. This allows it to be distinguished from other small related and similar-looking plants such as Mouse-ears (*Cerastium* spp.), which are hairy all over.

USES The name *chickweed* refers to its use as a feed to fatten up poultry. However, it is also a top edible herb for humans. It has a slight salty taste and is dense in minerals, nutrients and protein, and is therefore excellent for recovering convalescents. It is best used fresh in salads or use like you would spinach.

When taken internally, chickweed is demulcent on the gastric system, soothing irritated tissues in conditions like IBS and after gastric infection.

Externally, chickweed works wonders for a wide range of inflamed, itchy skin problems, from cuts to nettle stings, chickenpox, eczema, and psoriasis, and is a particularly gentle remedy for children. It is best used fresh: squeeze the juice onto itchy, hot rashes, or infuse in water and chill to make cooling compresses and baths. Alternatively, puréed chickweed can be mixed with aloe vera gel and frozen into ice cubes (see recipe on page 144), then applied to hot itchy skin conditions, or it can be added to smoothies for internal use.

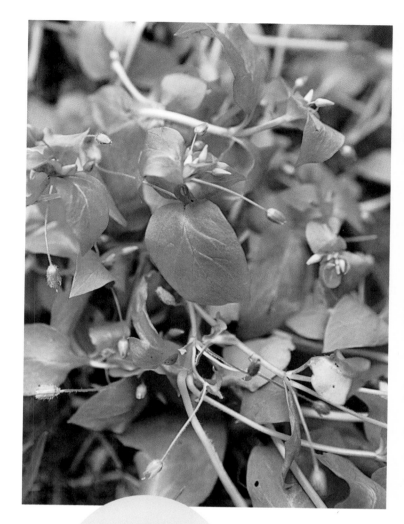

TIP
Freshly dried chickweed can be infused in oil and added to creams as a specific remedy for itchy eczema.

CHICKWEED AND ALOE COOLING CUBES

The anti-inflammatory and anti-itch properties of chickweed are combined with cooling aloe, to create handy-size ice cubes for cooling sunburn, rashes, and stings.

½ cup fresh aloe vera gel (see method)
2 handfuls of fresh chickweed

Slice the gel from the inner aloe leaves, taking care to discard the inner green and yellow leaf lining. Measure the gel (you need ½ cup), then put it into a blender with the chickweed and blend together until combined.

Alternatively, buy pre-mixed aloe vera gel and add to the blended chickweed.

Spoon into ice cube trays and freeze until solid.

To use, apply a frozen cube to the affected area, as and when needed.

SHELF LIFE Up to 1 year in the freezer.

CAUTION For external use only.

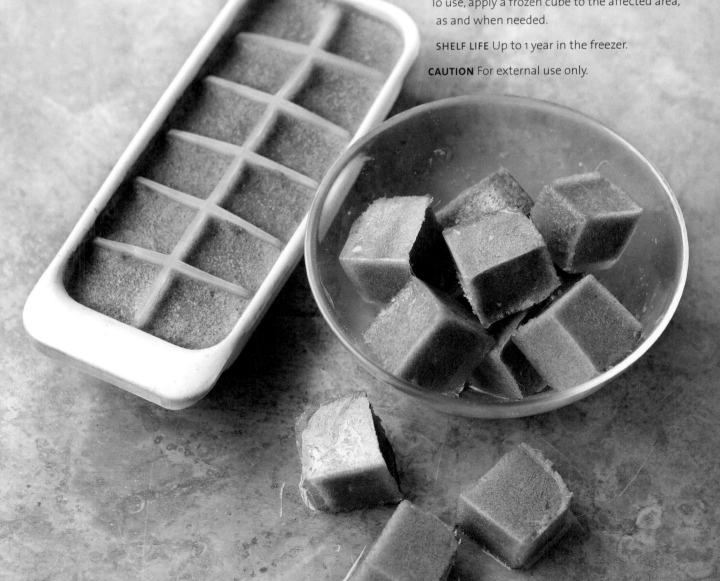

Symphytum spp.
Boraginaceae

COMMON NAME Comfrey

PARTS USED Leaves.

ACTIONS Vulnerary, demulcent, bone healing, tissue healing.

INDICATIONS Broken bones, fractures, shallow wounds, varicose ulcers, scar tissue.

DESCRIPTION The leaves are large and oval in shape with elegant, curving veins. The whole plant is covered in hairs, which some people find irritating. The texture of the leaves resembles an unshaven chin! This should distinguish it, when not in flower, from the potentially toxic but similar-looking foxglove, whose leaves are soft and velvety. The blue-purple flowers grow in a scorpiod cyme: a spiral-curl arranged like a snail shell.

There are many species of comfrey that can all be used for external use, but the official one is best and has a distinctive feature; the leaves grow in a "wing" that reaches down the stem all the way to the next leaf.

USES One of comfrey's old country names is "knitbone" and it is used for just that: to help heal broken bones. Its remarkable properties don't stop there, however; it is also beneficial for tendons, ligaments, and skin healing. It contains a compound called allantoin that encourages the replication of new cells and improves scar formation. It is so effective at healing tissues that care must be taken with deep wounds or it will heal over the top, potentially "sealing" in infection and causing an abscess. In those cases, use calendula with antimicrobial herbs to prevent infection first.

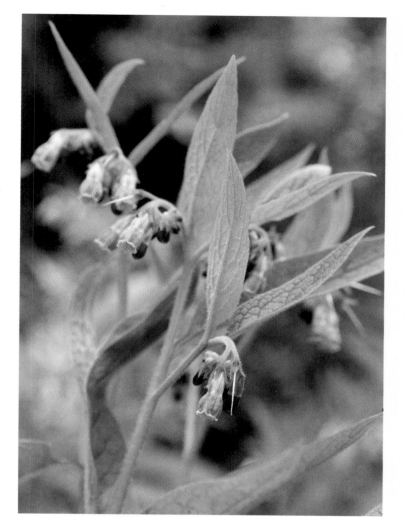

Traditionally, the leaf infusion was drunk for a maximum of six weeks for healing broken bones and stomach ulcers. However, this use has been discontinued by herbalists due to comfrey's content of chemicals called pyrrolizidine alkaloids, which can detrimentally affect liver health. Instead, use comfrey externally, as this is just as effective: apply it as a fresh leaf poultice or infuse newly dried leaves in oil to create rubs and balms. For broken bones and wounds, apply at least twice daily to the affected area for a maximum of 2 months.

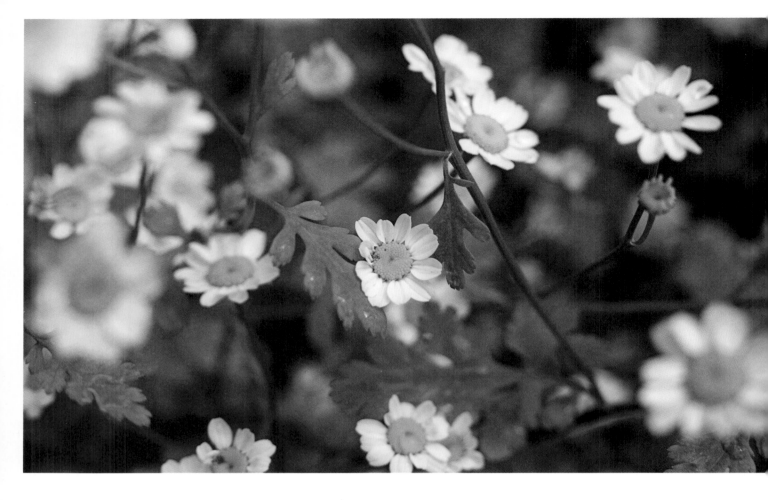

Tanacetum parthenium
Asteraceae

COMMON NAME Feverfew

PARTS USED Leaves and flowers.

ACTIONS Anti-inflammatory, anti-migraine, vasodilator, bitter.

INDICATIONS Migraines, headaches, tinnitus, dizziness, allergies.

DESCRIPTION Feverfew is an annual, daisy-looking plant; the flower has a yellow button center and white petals that grow in groups off the stem. It can grow knee-high and has an upright, stiff appearance. The leaves are lobed and a light matt green color.

USES Feverfew is an herbal medicine used specifically for headaches and migraines. It is bitter and circulatory in effect, and research has shown it inhibits inflammatory chemicals that can cause headaches and allergies. The leaves are traditionally taken fresh in butter because the constituents are made more bioavailable in fats. The dosage is one fresh leaf three times a day but can also be taken in tinctures. Feverfew can also be taken for tinnitus, vertigo and dizziness.

CAUTIONS Do not use in pregnancy, or with aspirin or anticoagulant medication.

Taraxacum officinale
Asteraceae

COMMON NAMES Dandelion, Wet-the-bed

PARTS USED Roots, leaves, flowers, latex.

ACTIONS Bitter, hepatic, kidney stimulant, laxative, diuretic.

INDICATIONS Constipation, water retention, poor appetite, rheumatism, and arthritis.

DESCRIPTION Popular childhood games of blowing dandelion's fluffy seed heads "to tell the time" or to make a wish are common around the world. Its bright yellow, multi-petaled flower resembles a lion's mane and its deeply cut leaves were also thought to be similar to the jagged teeth of a lion, hence the name being an Anglicized version of the French for "lion's teeth": *dent-de-lion*. There are many closely related species of dandelion; any that contain a white sap (latex) are also used medicinally.

USES There are numerous traditional uses recorded for this wonderful herb, probably because it grows everywhere, to the despair of many gardeners! Don't weed out your dandelions, though — embrace them! The roots can be roasted and ground to make a nice nutty, caffeine-free substitute for coffee. The sap was said to get rid of warts, but greater celandine (*Chelidonium majus*) is better for this. Use dandelion sap instead to make temporary tattoos: apply a design to the skin, avoid rubbing it off, and within a few hours it will have turned into a light brown marking.

Medicinally, the dandelion is associated with kidney and liver ailments. Traditionally, the leaf was used for increasing urine (hence its other name, wet-the-bed). The root was used for stimulating the liver and bile production; both can be used fairly interchangeably, however. Therefore it can be used as an infusion or tincture for urine infections, and herbalists use it for certain types of water retention associated with premenstrual syndrome and heart failure. Because it contains high levels of potassium, it does not cause a deficiency as some prescribed diuretics do.

The whole plant is bitter, particularly the root, which has digestive stimulating properties. This action can be harnessed in a decoction to encourage bowel movements (bile being a natural laxative) and is safe and effective, even for children. Dandelion aids the liver and kidneys to clear bodily wastes, and it is a go-to herb for those suffering from chronic skin problems including acne and eczema, and joint problems including arthritis and rheumatism.

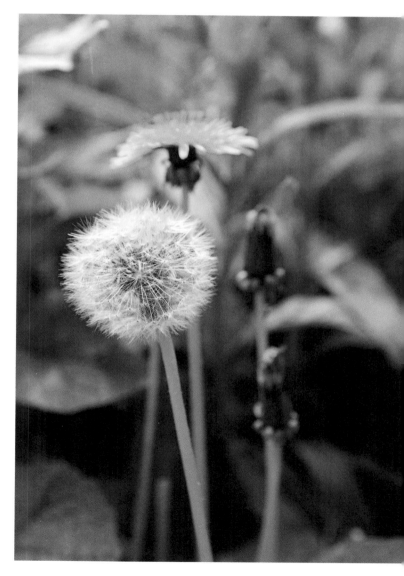

Trifolium pratense
Fabaceae

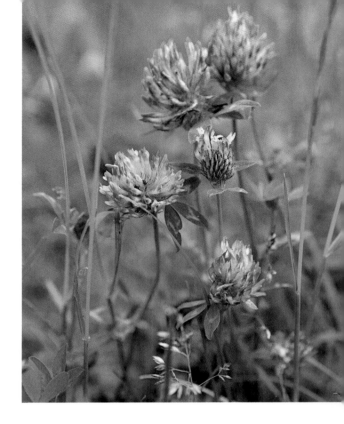

COMMON NAME Red Clover

PARTS USED Aerial parts.

ACTIONS Alterative, diuretic, expectorant, tonic.

INDICATIONS Chronic skin conditions, acne, eczema, psoriasis, menopausal hot flashes, hormonal imbalance.

DESCRIPTION This small, ground-covering plant can often be found in open fields and meadows. It's native to Europe, but naturalized in the United States and Australia. It fixes nitrogen in the ground to enrich the soil — hence the saying "to be in clover", i.e. to be rich. It has a compound leaf with three (or even four if you are lucky!) round or slightly pointed leaflets common to the whole clover family. The reddish-purple flowers are arranged in a globular head. It is fairly common, but there is also a lot of white clover found in lawns and meadows, which is not used medicinally. If you have found clover in your lawn and wonder which one it is before it has flowered, take a look at the underside of the leaf: the red variety will be hairy.

USES Herbalists use red clover for its gentle mineral-rich alterative and diuretic actions that influence the lymphatic system for clearing the lymph glands, breast tissue, and skin. Herbalists use it for painful breasts and armpits, particularly associated with hormonal issues. Its cleansing action means it is also used as a remedy for clearing troublesome skin problems such as acne, eczema, and psoriasis.

Red clover is famed for alleviating menopausal symptoms. It contains phytoestrogens that balance hormones and help to relieve hot flashes, breast pain, and irritability. Its high mineral content can help with bone density loss around menopause. Because of its gentle and steady action, it can be used over long periods of time to benefit from its therapeutic effects.

CLEANSING AND NOURISHING TEA

This tea is nourishing to the body and cleansing to the lymph glands. Use for painful breasts and skin problems.

1 ounce dried red clover flowers
1 ounce dried cleavers
1 ounce dried calendula flowers
1 ounce dried oat straw
1 ounce dried nettle leaves

Mix all the dried herbs together in a sterilized jar, then seal, label, and date.

To use, place 1 teaspoon of the dried herb mix in 1 cup of boiling water and leave to infuse for 15 minutes, then strain and drink.

Take up to three times a day, as and when needed.

SHELF LIFE The dried herb mix will keep in a cool, dark place for up to 1 year.

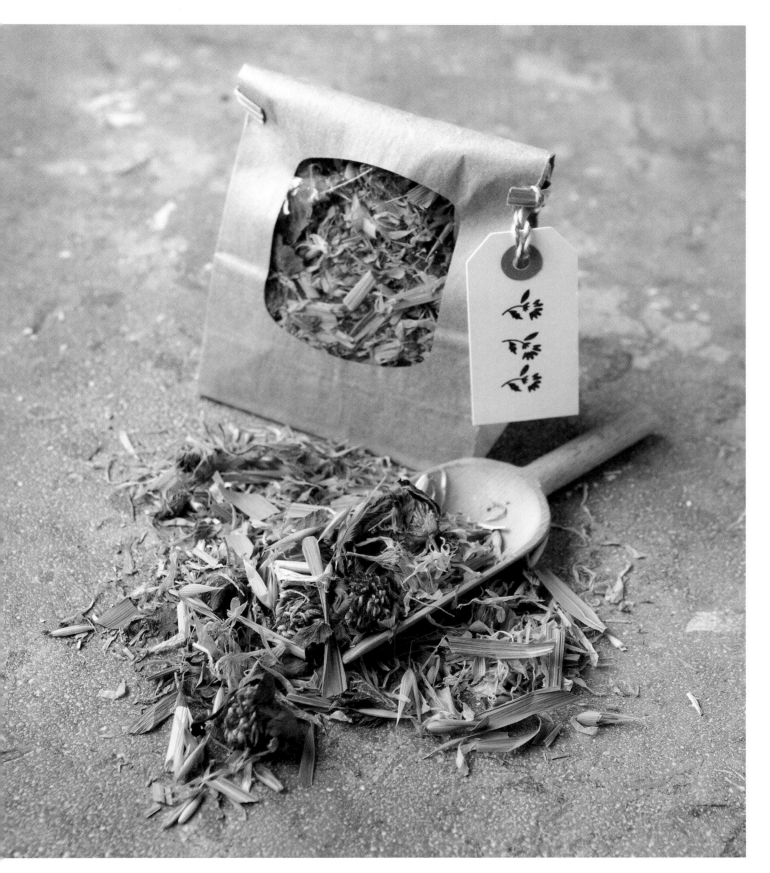

Urtica dioica
Urticaceae

COMMON NAMES Nettle, Stinging Nettle

PARTS USED Leaves, seeds, roots.

ACTIONS Nutritive, tonic, alterative, astringent, styptic, diuretic, adrenal tonic, anti-allergy.

INDICATIONS Anemia, stress, allergies, arthritis, eczema, convalescence, hair and nails, weak skin.

DESCRIPTION Culpeper, the 17th-century herbalist, wrote: "Nettles are so well known, that they need no description; they can be found by feeling, in the darkest night". The whole plant is covered in a fine layer of hairs, some containing formic acid and histamine that irritate the skin when touched. It is a perennial herb growing up to about 3 feet high, with heart-shaped, toothed leaves. The tiny greenish white flowers appear in summer on long dangling clusters like waterfalls.

Stinging nettles can vary in appearance depending on soil conditions — some mature leaves can have tinges of reddish purple, some are small, some large. There are also lots of nettle lookalikes, e.g. white dead-nettle and red or purple dead-nettle (*Lamium album* and *Lamium purpureum*). If in doubt, find out the Culpeper way; with touch!

HARVEST Use gloves to avoid the stinging hairs; some people find if they "grasp the nettle" firmly, they remain unbothered, but the latter option is only for the brave! Nettle tops (the top 2–3 sets of leaves) should be picked before the plant sets flower in late spring/early summer. After the nettle has flowered, uric acid crystals can form in the leaves; these can be irritating to the kidneys, so it's best to harvest the leaves before flowering. It's also best to harvest in spring or again in autumn when the nettle has a second flush. This can be encouraged with periodic cutting back. A trick to harvest the seeds is to hang the plant in paper bags upside down, dry for a few days, and then shake the bags to dislodge the seeds. Roots should be dug up in the autumn.

USES Nettle is known for its blood-nourishing, alterative, and blood-cleansing effects. It is a highly nutritious plant; its extensive root system draws up minerals from deep within the soil, making it rich in iron, calcium, selenium, zinc, magnesium, potassium, and other trace minerals. It contains many vitamins, including vitamins A and C, and is also high in protein and amino acids. It is an all-round "superfood". Add fresh nettles to juices, foods, and teas to help to improve hair, skin, and nail quality. For year-round use, keep a jar of dried nettle leaves in the kitchen to sprinkle into soups, stews, gravies and sauces to increase your mineral and nutrient intake — beware, though, the dried nettles can still sting, but will be rendered harmless with cooking.

Nettle is an all-round tonic herb,

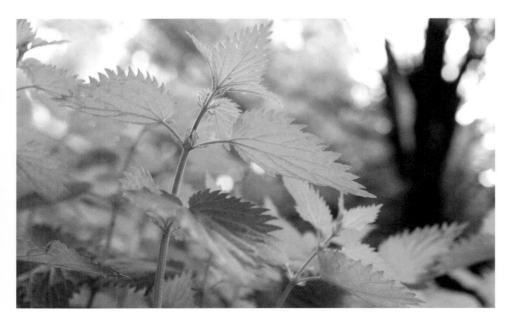

feeding the tissues and helping to keep the body in a state of vitality, improving energy, circulation, and mental clarity. The antihistamine effects of nettle make them helpful for the treatment of allergies such as hay fever and eczema. Use fresh or dried nettles in infusions or tinctures. Nettle infusion also makes a great final hair rinse to add shine and body to hair, and is used to treat dandruff (see the Hair Tonic recipe on page 74).

The seeds are used to support the adrenal glands, acting as an adaptogen to support the body in times of increased stress. Eat them fresh off the plant, freeze or tincture them, as they do not keep well once dried. Try the Energy Balls on page 66.

Nettle root is used by herbalists in the treatment of benign prostate enlargement and has promising research to support its use.

Verbascum thapsus
Scrophulariaceae

COMMON NAME Mullein

PARTS USED Flowers, leaves.

ACTIONS Demulcent, antimicrobial.

INDICATIONS Ear infections, bronchitis, catarrh, coughs.

DESCRIPTION Mullein is a biennial herb with a tall, strong, straight stem. It is covered in a thick coat of soft, silvery hairs, giving it a fuzzy appearance. The fluffy stems were once dipped in wax and used as candles, giving it the name "hag's tapers." The flowers are symmetrical, five-petaled and a pale golden yellow. Other species, including the black or dark mullein (*Verbascum nigrum*), which is less furry, can also be used medicinally.

USES Due to its soothing mucilaginous content and anti-microbial volatile oils, mullein's most common use is for healing and reducing the pain of infected ears, swollen

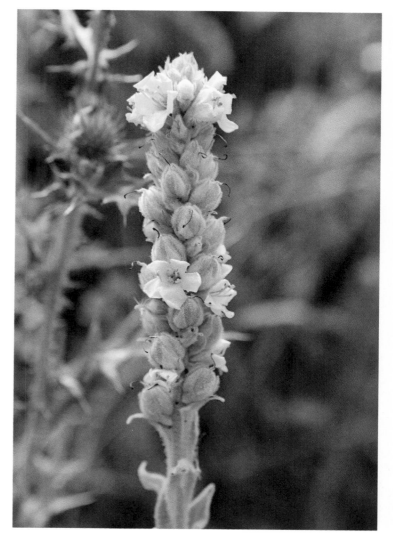

glands, and chesty coughs. An infused oil of the flowers can be placed in the outer ear using a cotton ball.
It combines well with other antimicrobial herbs, such as garlic or St John's wort–infused oil or a few drops of lavender essential oil, to help ease inflammation and pain.

Mullein can also be used to soothe both phlegmy and dry coughs. Take mullein internally in infusions or tinctures at the same time to support healing.

CAUTION Mullein oil should not be placed directly into the ear, especially in cases of perforated eardrum as this can cause infection.

Verbena officinalis
Verbenaceae

COMMON NAME Vervain

PARTS USED Leaves and flowers.

ACTIONS Nervine, antispasmodic, astringent, liver-protecting, menstrual tonic, diaphoretic.

INDICATIONS Anxiety, stress, menstrual pain, PMS, indigestion, colds, flu.

DESCRIPTION Vervain is a sweet and unassuming perennial plant with multiple knobbly flower spikes arising from the main stem. The tiny, pink to lavender-colored flowers circle the stem like little crowns. The leaves change from being toothed higher up to deeply lobed at the base and have a slight sandpapery feel to them. Lemon verbena, a popular herb for teas, is not the same plant, though it is related.

USES Vervain has a reputation as a magical plant and was revered as a panacea by many ancient civilizations, including the Greeks and Romans. It can be used fresh on grazes and hot infected cuts, but it is mainly used as an herb for steadying the nerves, particularly for stress, anxiety, and premenstrual tension. Because it has antispasmodic and liver-stimulating actions, it helps to balance and clear hormones and soothe menstrual pain. The antispasmodic action can also help to ease digestive cramps. Vervain can also be taken as a hot infusion for its diaphoretic properties to encourage sweating in fevers such as for colds and flu.

CAUTION Avoid in pregnancy.

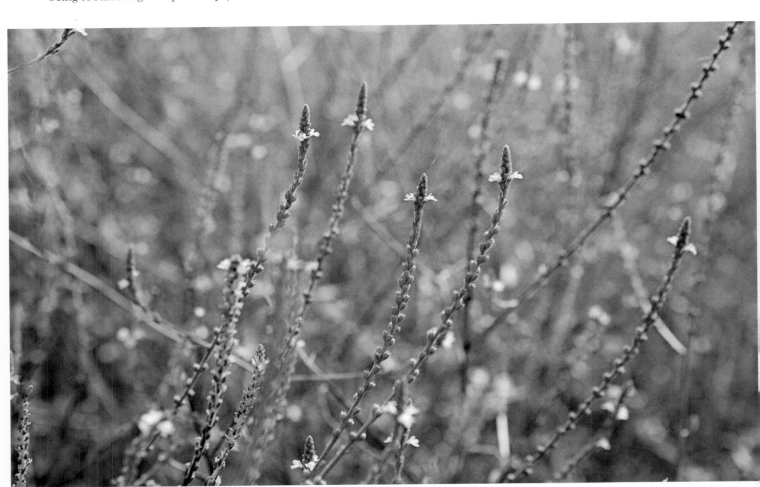

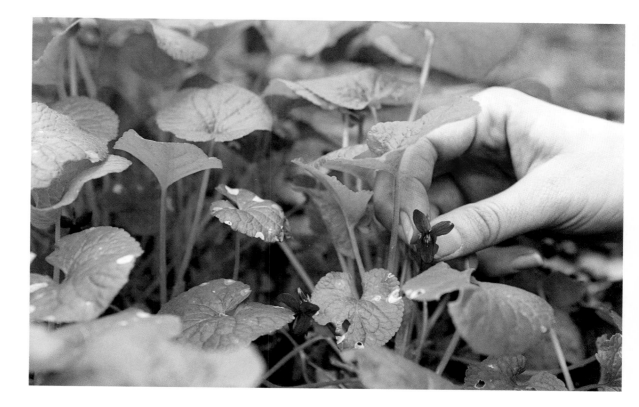

Viola spp. (V. odorata)
Violaceae

COMMON NAME Sweet Violet

PARTS USED Leaves and flowers.

ACTIONS Demulcent, circulatory, vein strengthening.

INDICATIONS Eczema, bruises, circulatory, coughs.

DESCRIPTION Violets prefer to grow in areas of dappled shade, where their nodding purple flowers shine in undergrowth like little gems. Take a sniff — their delicate scent is distinctively sweet and gives the species V. odorata its name, distinguishing it from the scentless dog violet (V. riviniana). Their dark green leaves are heart-shaped and only a little larger than your thumb. They are becoming more rare to find, so, as with all plants you are interested in, please think of cultivating them if you would like to learn more.

USES Violets have been used to scent confectionery and make an attractive edible flower, either used fresh in salads or crystallized for use on cakes. In the celebrated Italian medieval medicinal school at Salerno, they were revered to dispel drunkenness and migraines. However, in modern herbal medicine, because the leaves are high in antioxidant and vein- and skin-strengthening rutin, they are used for skin disorders. Use in infusions, tinctures and creams for eczema, to help strengthen vein walls, heal bruises, and improve circulation.

CAUTION Should be avoided by those with an allergy to salicylic acid.

TIP To make crystallized violet flowers, paint each flower with whipped egg white. Lay out on wax paper and dust with powdered sugar. Leave to dry for 24 hours.

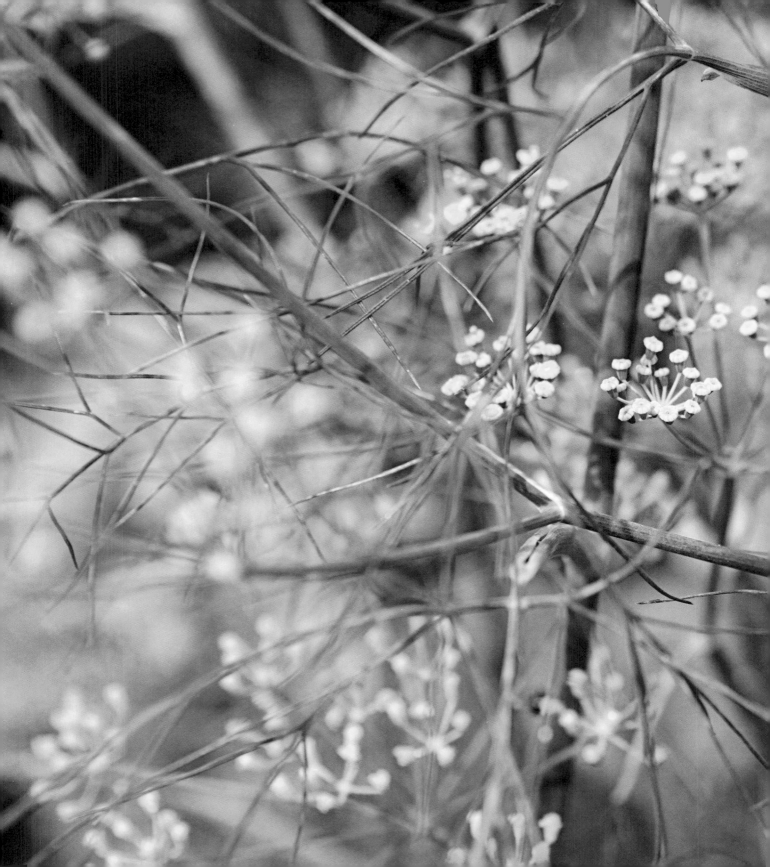

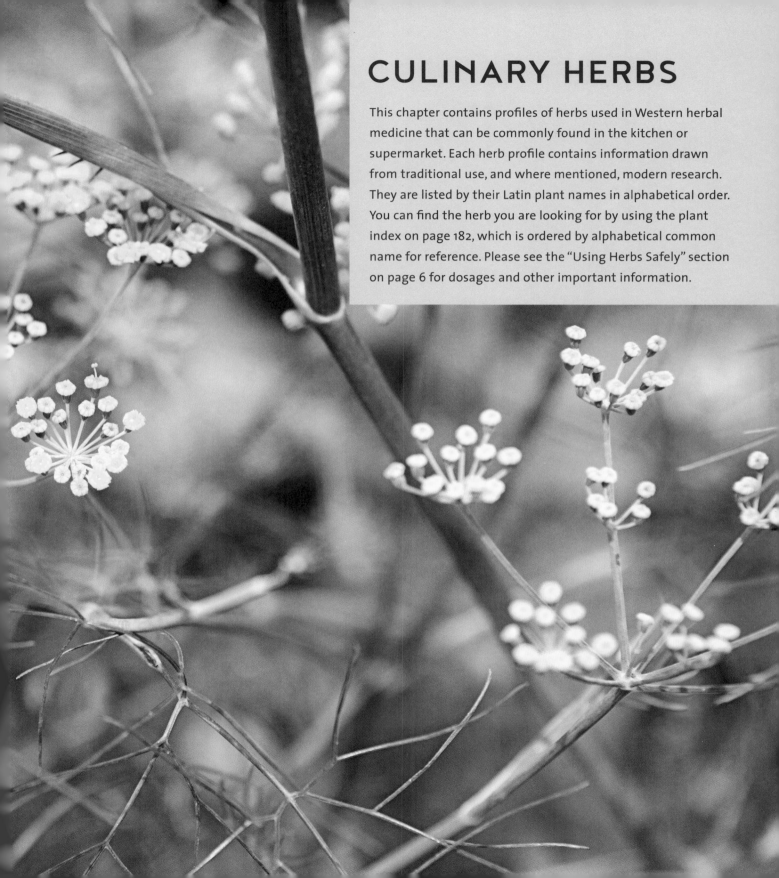

CULINARY HERBS

This chapter contains profiles of herbs used in Western herbal medicine that can be commonly found in the kitchen or supermarket. Each herb profile contains information drawn from traditional use, and where mentioned, modern research. They are listed by their Latin plant names in alphabetical order. You can find the herb you are looking for by using the plant index on page 182, which is ordered by alphabetical common name for reference. Please see the "Using Herbs Safely" section on page 6 for dosages and other important information.

Many of the herbs that we use in cooking contain some form of volatile oil; this is what gives them their aroma and what makes them taste so delicious. Culinary herbs not only bring flavor to the table, they are also powerful medicines in their own right. The volatile oils that infuse our dishes with flavor are potent antimicrobials. In times before modern refrigeration, they would act to preserve food. This is why in hot countries, food is often prepared with more herbs and spices.

With the invention of refrigeration and synthetic preservatives, convenience foods high in fat, salt, and sugar have become the staple flavorings of today. The full healing potential of culinary herbs has been forgotten and we often think of them as merely seasonings.

Not only are herbs rich in real flavor, they are high in phytochemicals that prevent illness and encourage vitality. They act to stimulate digestion, allowing us to process the nutrients from our food more efficiently. Culinary herbs are great preventative herbs; many have traditional uses as tonics and for longevity. Being high in antimicrobial volatile oils, they also make effective remedies for acute illness, making them perfect for everyday ailments and minor emergencies, as the chances are you will have something on hand in the kitchen to combat your ills.

Use culinary herbs regularly in the diet and cook from scratch where possible. If time for cooking is an issue, cook one-pot, herb-rich soups, sauces, and stews in bulk and freeze them in individual portions for later use. To get the most from culinary herbs, include them daily in the diet. In terms of dosage, they tend to be well tolerated, so use 1–3 teaspoons of fresh or dried herbs to each portion of food you prepare. Sprinkle freshly cut/chopped herbs into salads and over soups, rice, and stews, or make them into teas and tinctures and take in doses outlined on pages 157–165.

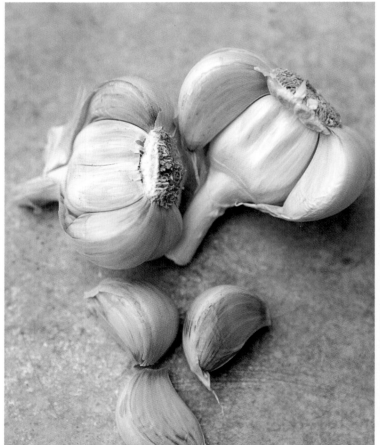
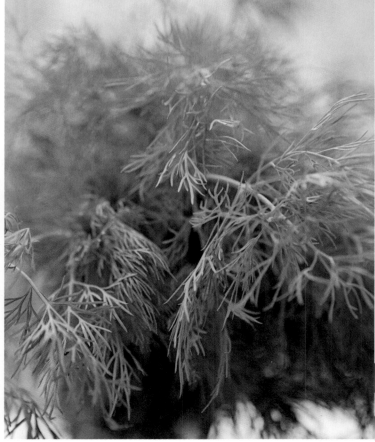

Allium sativum
Garlic

ACTIONS Antiviral, antimicrobial, antifungal, antioxidant, hypotensive.

INDICATIONS Colds, flu, coughs, bronchitis, gastric infections, high blood pressure, high cholesterol.

A very effective at-home remedy for chest infections and bronchitis is to crush a garlic clove and mix it with 2 tablespoons of honey. Take 1 teaspoon every few hours.

The smell of garlic comes from its content of sulfur-rich compounds, which are largely excreted through the lungs, giving the characteristic "garlic breath" after eating it. These sulfur compounds are highly antimicrobial and therefore act as powerful healers in respiratory infections.

Garlic has potent antioxidant properties; when taken regularly it has been shown to lower cholesterol and protect blood vessel walls, reducing the risk of hardening of the arteries and heart disease.

The best way to use garlic is daily, in food. It is most potent when used raw. The sulfur compounds (particularly allicin) in garlic are released after the membranes of the bulbs are damaged, so crush cloves 5 minutes before use to allow these compounds to develop. Aim to have 1–2 cloves a day. Chewing parsley or drinking milk after eating garlic can help reduce garlic breath.

CAUTION Those taking blood-thinning drugs should not suddenly increase garlic quantity in the diet.

Anethum graveolens
Dill

ACTIONS Carminative, digestive.

INDICATIONS Gastric discomfort, flatulence, colic.

Dill is one of the gentlest carminative herbs, making it useful even for colic in babies. A weak infusion of the seeds or herb can be given directly to infants, or taken in normal strength infusions by nursing mothers to pass the therapeutic effects through the breast milk.

Brassica alba, B. nigra
Mustard Seed

ACTIONS Warming, circulatory stimulant, digestive.

INDICATIONS Coughs, colds, flu, sinus congestion, chills, muscle pain, sluggish digestion.

Infused mustard oil makes a great warming massage rub for cold days and aching muscles. When digestion is sluggish, massage the tummy with the infused oil or add a dollop of mustard to food to stimulate digestion and relieve wind.

MUSTARD FOOTBATH

For tired feet, coughs, colds, and stuffy sinuses, try a mustard footbath. Fill a large bowl with comfortably hot water and sprinkle in 2 teaspoons of mustard powder. Soak the feet for 20 minutes while relaxing. When used in this way, mustard increases circulation to the feet, drawing congestion away from the head, relieving the pressure and inflammation that causes discomfort.

Capsicum spp.
Chile, Chile Pepper

Capsicum frutescens
Hot Pepper, Cayenne Pepper

ACTIONS Warming, circulatory stimulant, analgesic, diaphoretic, counter-irritant, antiseptic.

INDICATIONS Arthritis, myalgia, poor circulation, neuralgia, sinus congestion.

Chiles are incredibly heating. If you have ever had a spicy curry, you will be familiar with their warming and diaphoretic effects. The best way to take chile is in food; it stimulates and heats the digestion, assisting the assimilation of nutrients and the medicinal effects of other herbs. Take chile for congestion; it will help clear mucus from the head, sinuses and lungs. It encourages blood flow to the extremities for those who suffer from cold hands and feet or have a cold constitution in general.

A pinch of chile powder and salt in a hot chocolate or added to Golden Milk (see recipe on page 65) is an indulgent and delicious way to take chiles; the fat in the milk also mutes the burning heat, so those who cannot have spicy foods can tolerate higher amounts.

Chile-infused oil can be massaged onto sore muscles and rheumatic joints to lessen pain. This may seem counterintuitive, to increase blood flow to an already inflamed area. However, increased circulation can aid in the clearance of inflammatory chemicals and reduce swelling. Chiles also contain capsaicin, a phytochemical that reduces substance P, a pain transmitter in the nerves. This has been found to reduce pain, especially in chronic conditions such as rheumatism, arthritis, and sciatica.

CAUTION When using chiles, do not touch eyes; wash hands well after use.

Cinnamomum zeylanicum
Cinnamon

ACTIONS Carminative, antiemetic, antimicrobial, warming, diaphoretic, circulatory stimulant.

INDICATIONS Gastric infections, nausea, colds, flu, high cholesterol.

Cinnamon is a warming and drying herb; use it for colds and flu to "dry" and clear mucus from the lungs and sinuses and to break a fever. It encourages blood circulation to the digestive system and extremities, warming cold hands and feet and igniting digestive fire in those with a weak gut. Cinnamon has slightly astringent actions and is antimicrobial; a hot infusion with honey and lemon can reduce diarrhea and nausea caused by gastric infections.

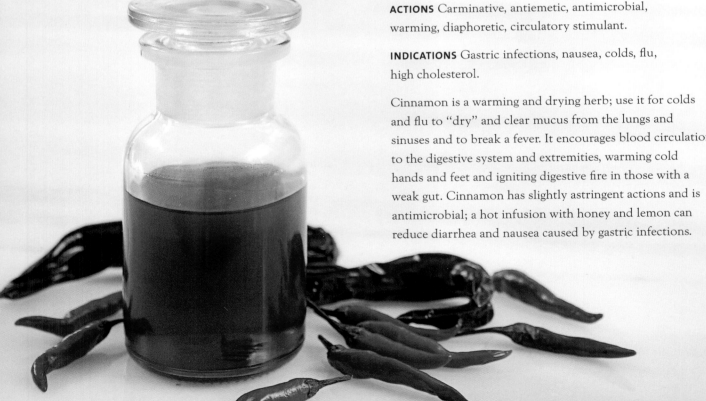

Curcuma longa
Turmeric

ACTIONS Anti-inflammatory, antioxidant, alterative, anti-arthritic, hepatoprotective, immune modulator, antiviral, cholesterol-lowering.

INDICATIONS Skin infections, acne, eczema, gastric inflammation, joint inflammation, arthritis, aging.

Turmeric has been used throughout Asia for millennia, with mention of the herb dating as far back as four thousand years. Traditionally, turmeric was used as an digestive and a herb for longevity. It is highly antioxidant and recent research has shown that turmeric can lessen the effects of oxidation damage to tissues throughout the body. Use it to reduce inflammation in chronic conditions such as arthritis and rheumatism, and inflammatory skin conditions.

Turmeric has a tonic effect on the circulatory system; it thins the blood, protects the blood vessels, and has been shown to lower cholesterol. It has a pungent, bitter taste, which stimulates the liver and digestive system, aiding the digestive process and allowing for the efficient assimilation of nutrients from the food we eat.

Use a teaspoon of freshly grated turmeric or turmeric powder daily in cooking, add to Golden Milk (see page 65), or make up a batch of the Turmeric Anti-inflammatory Balls (right). Adding a pinch of black pepper when taking turmeric assists the bioavailability of its anti-inflammatory compounds, as does taking turmeric with fat-based products such as milk or coconut oil.

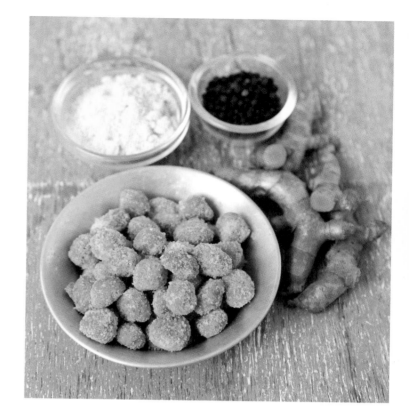

TURMERIC ANTI-INFLAMMATORY BALLS

Based loosely on a traditional Ayurvedic preparation of turmeric and honey, these balls are an easy and tasty way to get turmeric and its anti-inflammatory effects into the diet. You can also use freshly grated turmeric.

2 teaspoons high-quality turmeric powder
1 tablespoon set/thick honey
½ teaspoon freshly ground black pepper
2 tablespoons ground almonds, plus extra for dusting
1 teaspoon coconut oil

Put all the ingredients into a bowl and mix together to form a stiff paste.

Roll the mixture into balls about the size of a chickpea and then coat with a dusting of ground almonds. Store in an airtight container in the fridge.

To use, take 1–2 balls daily. **SHELF LIFE** Up to 1 month in the fridge.

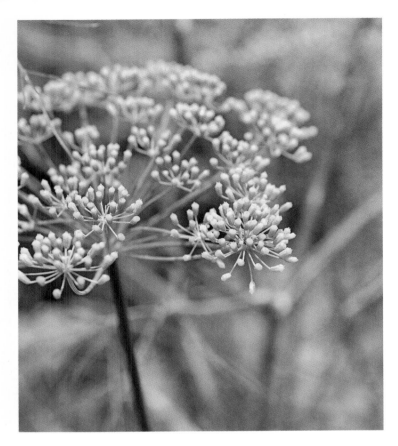

Foeniculum vulgare
Fennel Seed

ACTIONS Antimicrobial, carminative, galactagogue.

INDICATIONS Flatulence, poor digestion, bloating, poor lactation.

Fennel is an herb with ancient use; it is mentioned as one of nine sacred herbs in an Anglo-Saxon herbal text, the Lacnunga. Today, fennel is primarily a digestive herb. Its aromatic and warming qualities reduce cramping and bloating, and dispel wind in the gut.

It is a gentle herb that can be used even for infant colic as a weak infusion by the teaspoonful. Alternatively, nursing mothers can drink the tea as the therapeutic properties are passed on through breast milk. It also stimulates breast milk production where lactation is scanty or delayed.

Glycyrrhiza glabra
Licorice

ACTIONS Expectorant, demulcent, adaptogen, adrenal tonic, anti-inflammatory.

INDICATIONS Coughs, colds, flu, adrenal fatigue, convalescence, gastric infection, gastritis, irritable bowel, skin irritation, eczema, hormonal disruption.

Licorice contains plant glycosides that act similarly to the precursors of some of the body's natural endocrine hormones. It has an adaptogenic tonic effect on the endocrine glands, making it a useful addition to herbal mixes for many kinds of hormonal disorders, including polycystic ovarian syndrome (PCOS) and adrenal fatigue. It has a specific affinity for the adrenal glands, supporting their function in times of increased stress.

Glycyrrhizin, a compound in licorice, gives it a sweet taste; it is fifty times sweeter than sugar. Added to herbal blends that contain bitter plants, liquorice's sweetness improves palatability.

Licorice is expectorant, demulcent and immune-boosting, helping to clear mucus from the chest in colds and flu and soothe inflamed tissues. Its demulcent effects extend to the gut, where it has earned itself a reputation for healing ulcers and calming irritable bowel disease and gastritis. Licorice can be added to creams to soothe irritated skin and eczema externally too.

CAUTION High doses of licorice over prolonged periods may cause a rise in blood pressure and is contraindicated with blood pressure medications.

Mentha spp.
Mints

ACTIONS Cooling, carminative, antispasmodic.

INDICATIONS Headaches, colds, flu, flatulence, nausea.

Mints are a soothing and cooling remedy. For hot, pounding headaches and stuffy sinuses, massage one drop of peppermint essential oil diluted in a few drops of base oil over the temples and forehead. Alternatively, shred fresh mint leaves into a bowl and pour over boiling water for an airway clearing steam.

Combined with yarrow and elderflower, peppermint is a traditional tea for colds and flu. Drink a cup of fresh mint tea after a large meal to lessen bloating. Peppermint tea eases upset stomachs and is a great remedy for vomiting. Its pleasant taste means it is often well tolerated by children.

CAUTION Do not use in cases of heartburn.

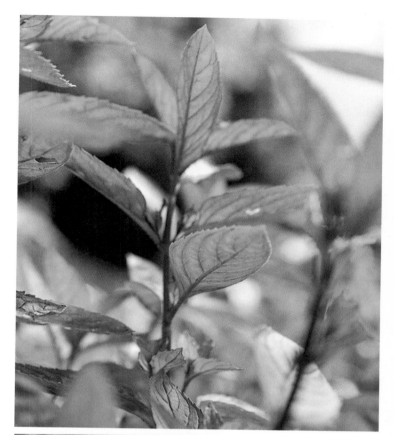

Ocimum basilicum
Basil

ACTIONS Antimicrobial, diaphoretic, circulatory stimulant.

INDICATIONS Infections, coughs, colds, flu, sinus inflammation, poor memory, stress, poor appetite, low vitality, convalescence.

Basil is an herb for the head — it improves circulation and soothes headaches, especially when caused by stress. Just the smell of freshly crushed basil leaves is uplifting to the spirits and stimulating to the appetite, making it a good herb for convalescents. In Ayurvedic medicine, tulsi or holy basil (*Ocimum tenuiflorum, O. sanctum*) has been used for centuries as a longevity herb, adaptogen, and cure-all. Like rosemary, basil is thought to stimulate circulation to the brain and improve memory. All types of aromatic basil have antimicrobial volatile oils that can be employed to treat sinus and respiratory infections in steam inhalations.

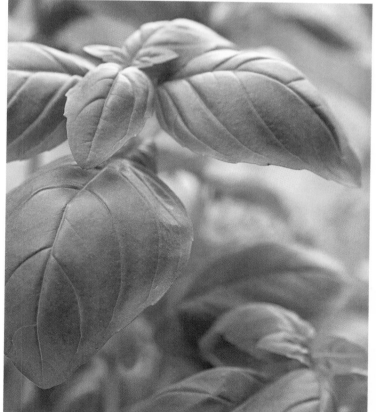

Origanum majorana
Sweet Marjoram

Origanum vulgare
Oregano/Wild Marjoram

ACTIONS Antibacterial, warming, expectorant.

INDICATIONS Muscle pain, rheumatism, thrush, fungal skin infections, fungal nails.

Both oregano and marjoram are used very similarly in medicine and cooking and can be used interchangeably. They both dry well and retain their aroma; in fact, the taste becomes sweeter when dried.

For muscle pain and rheumatism, use the infused oil or diluted essential oil of oregano as a warming, tension-easing massage. The volatile oils in oregano are highly antimicrobial; use the fresh, crushed herb or essential oil in a steam inhalation for colds and sinus infections, as it acts as an expectorant to remove phlegm. Drink the hot tea with honey for respiratory infections, bronchitis, and excess catarrh.

Dilute the tincture with water at a ratio of 1:2 and apply to fungal nails daily, or blend 20 drops of oregano essential oil in 2 teaspoons of base oil and massage into the infected nails. Add the essential oil or infused oil of oregano to cream blends for fungal skin infections.

For vaginal thrush, a strong tea can be added to a bath or used as a wash. For oral thrush, drink oregano infusion or gargle with the diluted tincture.

Petroselinum crispum
Parsley

ACTIONS Diuretic, emmenagogue, alterative, carminative.

INDICATIONS Anemia, scanty periods, gastric irritation, garlic breath.

Parsley is a nutritional powerhouse. It contains more iron than spinach and is high in other essential minerals, vitamins A and C, and antioxidant flavonoids, making it much more than just a garnish. It was traditionally regarded as an alterative "blood-building herb", used in convalescence and menstrual problems to bring on delayed menstruation. For this reason, it is best avoided in large quantities during pregnancy.

It is an aromatic herb that can be added to food to support weak digestion and lessen flatulence. Chew parsley after eating garlic as its volatile oils prevent garlic breath.

It has a diuretic effect and makes a useful addition to teas for urinary infections and water retention.

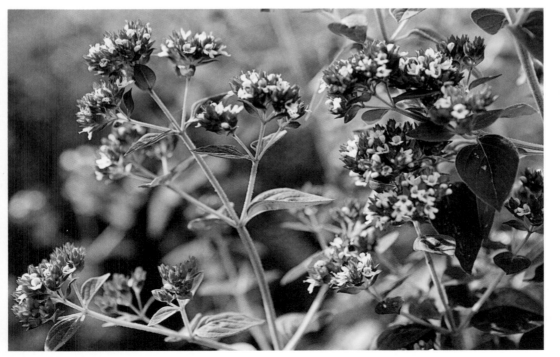

Rosmarinus officinalis
Rosemary

ACTIONS Warming, circulatory stimulant, diaphoretic, antioxidant, antimicrobial, carminative.

INDICATIONS Studying, poor concentration and memory, low mood, headaches, anxiety, sinus congestion, longevity, tiredness, dull complexion, thinning hair, dandruff, muscle pain, rheumatism, arthritis, debility, cystitis, sluggish digestion.

Rosemary has long been regarded as a longevity herb, thought to strengthen the mind and body and reinvigorate the sick and aging. It stimulates the circulatory system and encourages blood flow to the brain to relieve headaches that are caused by insufficient blood flow.

Rosemary is traditionally associated with remembrance, probably because of its memory-enhancing effects. It was once woven into garlands at weddings and worn on clothing at funerals. Use rosemary essential oil in a burner, or dilute in a base oil and rub on the temples and pulse points when studying or working for long periods, to improve mental clarity and calm the nerves. The main qualities of rosemary are stimulating and warming, and the aroma is uplifting to the mood.

The volatile oils present in rosemary are highly antimicrobial. For blocked sinuses, try a steam inhalation of rosemary, using either a few drops of the essential oil in boiling water or a strong infusion of the fresh herb.

An infused oil of rosemary eases aching muscles and joints when used in massage.

Added to face creams, rosemary brightens the complexion and stimulates circulation, reducing fatigued skin.

ROSEMARY HAIR OIL

Try infusing coconut oil with fresh rosemary (see page 24 for making oil infusions) for a scalp treatment to treat thinning hair and dandruff; it encourages growth and makes hair more lustrous and shiny. Add rosemary essential oil (up to 20 drops in 1/2 oil) for an extra boost. Simply massage it into the scalp and hair, then leave for 1 hour or up to overnight before washing off.

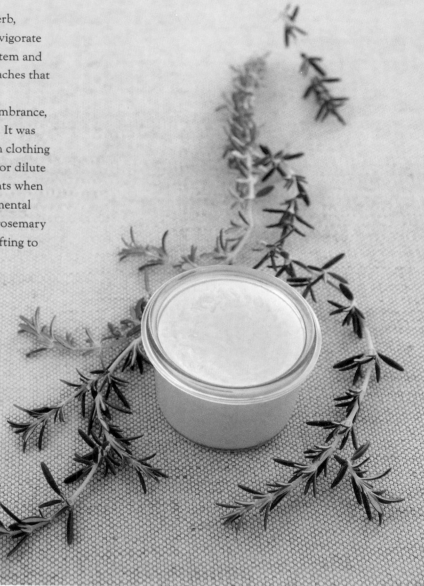

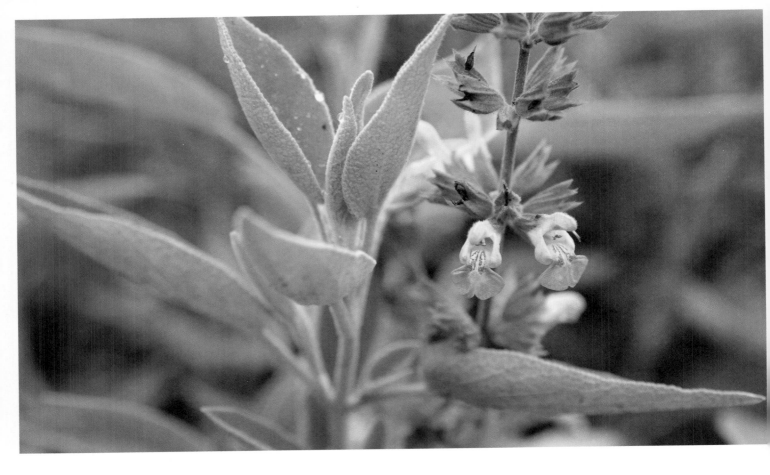

Salvia officinalis
Sage

ACTIONS Antimicrobial, astringent, antihydrotic, carminative, emmenagogue.

INDICATIONS Sore throats, gum disease, mouth ulcers, digestive discomfort, gastric infections, poor memory, aging, weaning, sweating, menopausal hot flashes.

Sage has a plethora of medicinal uses and was regarded as a panacea. A medieval proverb reads: "Why should a man die while sage grows in his garden."

Probably the most famous use of sage is in the treatment of menopausal night sweats. It is an astringent herb, reducing excess sweating and bodily secretions; it can also be used to dry up the breast milk of lactating mothers when weaning.

Sage is the traditional remedy for inflammations of the mouth and throat; it tones irritated tissues and kills bacteria. For mouth ulcers, sore gums, and sore throats, use it as a gargle in the form of a strong infusion or a diluted sage vinegar. Before toothbrushes became commonplace, the fresh leaves of sage were used to clean the teeth and strengthen the gums.

Sage is another of the aromatic herbs prized for its effects on the brain and memory; it contains powerful antioxidants that are known to combat the aging of cells. The terms "old sage" and "sage advice" say it all.

CAUTION Sage should be avoided in large quantities during pregnancy.

Thymus vulgaris
Thyme

ACTIONS Antimicrobial, antiviral, astringent, carminative, expectorant.

INDICATIONS Bronchitis, coughs, colds, flu, sinusitis, sore throats, asthma, toothache, cold sores, shingles, fungal skin infections, fungal nails, urinary infections.

Thyme is a pungent, powerfully antimicrobial herb. Its volatile oils are particularly antiviral and antifungal and are employed to treat urinary infections, skin infections, and fungal nails. Thyme acts as an expectorant, encouraging the removal of catarrh from the respiratory tract, and is useful in coughs and colds where there is lots of mucus present. It stimulates the immune system and strengthens the lungs.

For people who suffer from recurrent respiratory infections and mild asthma, drink a cup of thyme tea daily or eat a spoonful of thyme honey.

Thymol, a volatile oil in thyme, has anaesthetic and antimicrobial effects. Chew fresh thyme leaves to relieve the pain of toothache and inhibit the bacteria that cause infection.

CAUTION The essential oil of thyme is particularly potent and should be diluted well if applying to the skin. Do not use thyme in large quantities during pregnancy.

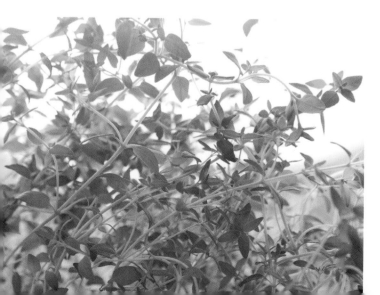

Zea mays
Corn Silk

ACTIONS Diuretic, anti-inflammatory, astringent, demulcent.

INDICATIONS Bladder infections, bladder inflammation.

If you have experienced the burning sensation of a urinary tract infection, you will know the desperation felt to ease the pain. When you need an emergency remedy, look to corn silk, the silky hairs that sit between the cob and the husk on an ear of sweetcorn. Corn silk infusions are demulcent, diuretic, and anti-inflammatory, helping to ease pain and flush out bacteria from the bladder. Use with urinary antiseptic herbs, such as thyme, juniper, and echinacea.

Zingiber officinale
Ginger

ACTIONS Antiemetic, carminative, anti-inflammatory, antimicrobial, circulatory stimulant, expectorant.

INDICATIONS Colds, flu, sinus infections, poor circulation, arthritis, colic, nausea, diarrhea, weak digestion, painful periods.

Ginger is the best herbal remedy for nausea and vomiting. A simple infusion, sipped in small amounts throughout the day, can lessen the nauseating effects of motion sickness, morning sickness and gastric upsets. Its antimicrobial effects also help kill off diarrhea- and vomiting-causing bacteria. Ginger strengthens and stimulates those with a weak digestion, especially in convalescence and the elderly.

Principally, ginger is a warming herb, lending its heating qualities to cold conditions. In colds, flu, and sinus infections, it aids in the clearance of phlegm and induces sweating to clear a fever. It stimulates the circulation, improving the supply of blood to the extremities, warming cold hands, feet, and arthritic conditions. Use it internally as a tea or externally as an infused oil.

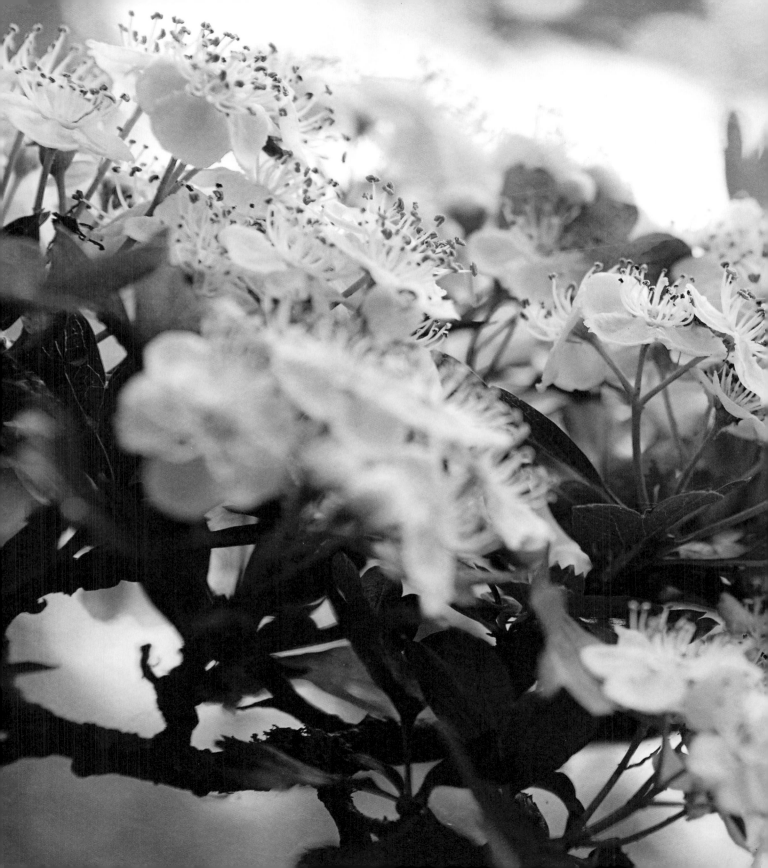

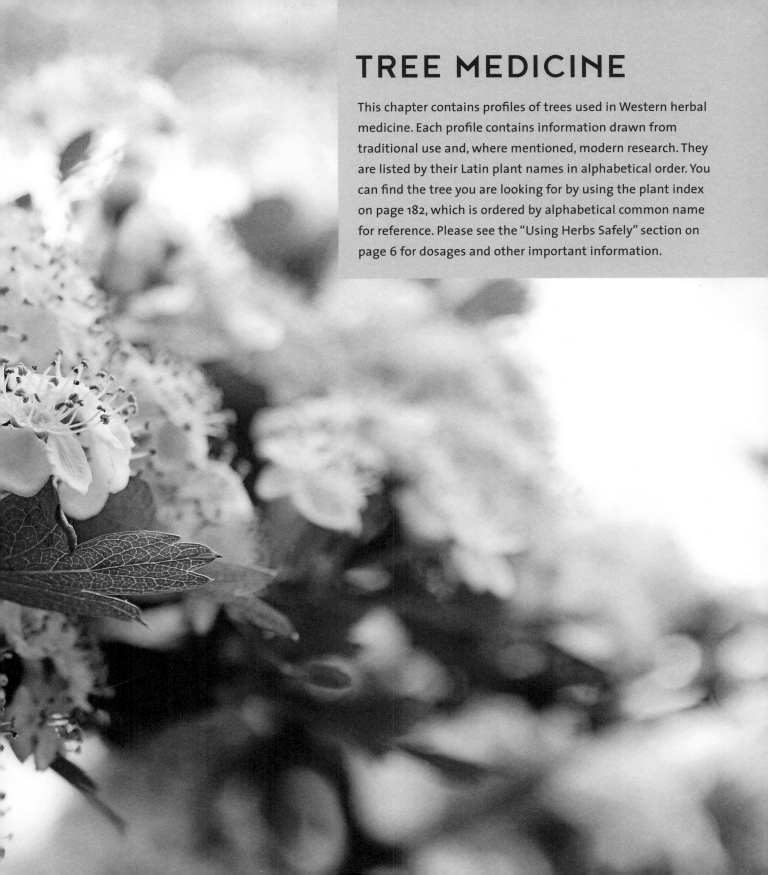

TREE MEDICINE

This chapter contains profiles of trees used in Western herbal medicine. Each profile contains information drawn from traditional use and, where mentioned, modern research. They are listed by their Latin plant names in alphabetical order. You can find the tree you are looking for by using the plant index on page 182, which is ordered by alphabetical common name for reference. Please see the "Using Herbs Safely" section on page 6 for dosages and other important information.

Aesculus hippocastanum, A. x *carnea*
Hippocastanaceae

COMMON NAMES Horse Chestnut, Red Horse Chestnut, Conker

PARTS USED Young leaves, bark, seeds, and seed capsules.

ACTIONS Vein strengthening, circulatory, astringent.

INDICATIONS Varicose veins, spider veins, hemorrhoids, poor circulation, sprains, cellulite, rosacea.

DESCRIPTION A tall deciduous tree bearing large, palmately compound leaves. Its small white or pink flowers are borne on spikes that look like candles and give this tree its other name of candelabra tree. Its large, shiny brown seeds, known as conkers, are protected by spiky green capsules.

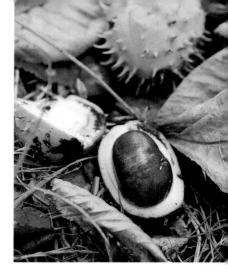

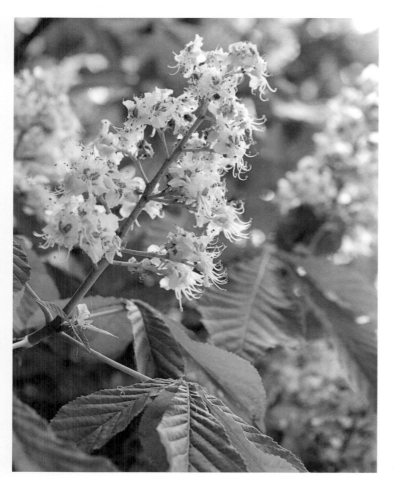

USES A favorite childhood pastime is to collect conkers by the bucket load in the hope of winning conker championships: a game where conkers are hung on strings and bashed at each other with the aim of breaking up their opponent's seed.

Horse chestnut is also a fantastic medicine; it tones and improves the venous circulation and is therefore a beneficial treatment for varicose veins and hemorrhoids. It is held in such high regard that in the past people believed that merely carrying conkers in your pocket would prevent bulging veins.

It is excellent in lotions and creams applied externally to problem veins, piles, achy muscles, and sprains. An infused oil of horse chestnut seed or leaf (when used externally) is also beneficial for reducing the appearance of cellulite and rosacea.

Collect conkers when just ripe (shiny and brown). The easiest way to process these very hard seeds is to place them in a clean pillowcase and break them open using a hammer. Then they are ready for tincturing and infusing in oil.

DOSAGE Although horse chestnut may be taken internally as a tincture, it can be irritating to sensitive stomachs and should be taken in low doses. Maximum ½ – ¾ teaspoon tincture per day. It is best used externally in cream or lotion 2–3 times a day.

CAUTION Should be avoided by pregnant and lactating women, and those with digestive ulcers.

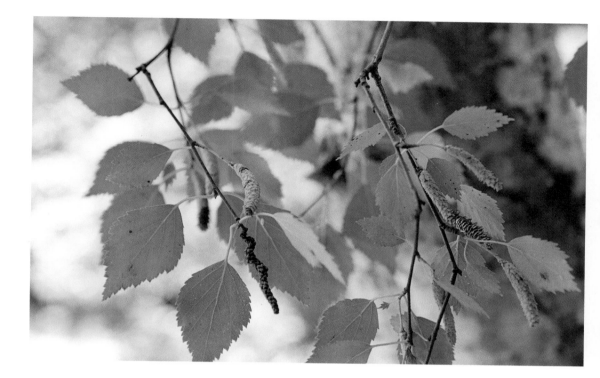

Betula pendula
Betulaceae

COMMON NAME Silver Birch

PARTS USED Young leaves, twigs, sap.

ACTIONS Diuretic, anti-inflammatory, astringent, diaphoretic, hypocholesterolemic.

INDICATIONS Cystitis, eczema, psoriasis, arthritis, rheumatism, high cholesterol, cellulite.

DESCRIPTION The defining feature of this tree is the papery silver-white bark that peels off from the trunk. The leaves are diamond-shaped and the branches sometimes hang in an elegantly weeping manner. The Downy Birch (*B. pubescens*) is a similar species with darker bark and downy twigs and can also be used medicinally.

USES Birch trees have long been used by people in northern climes for materials, medicine, and food. The papery bark has been used to write on, or made into tinder, hats, shoes, baskets, and boats, but today, it is often only chosen for gardens for its attractive bark and form. However, it has a wide range of medicinal uses that can be used at home.

The young leaves and twigs can be harvested and dried to use in infusions as a diuretic drink, beneficial for cystitis and urinary infections. The diuretic action has a cleansing and clearing effect on the body, so is useful for clearing inflammation and waste build-up for conditions such as rheumatism, arthritis, and chronic skin conditions. It has lipid-lowering and antioxidant effects that are thought to reduce high blood cholesterol. The young leaves can also be infused in oil and used externally to ease aching muscles and joints and improve the appearance of cellulite.

The sap is tapped in early spring as it rises, ready to awaken the tree from winter. It is most copious at this time and needs to be carefully harvested without killing the tree. However, it is becoming a popular beverage and can now be found in health food stores. Birch sap is high in fructose and is also diuretic, so can be used for similar conditions as the leaves.

CAUTION Not suitable for people sensitive to salicylates.

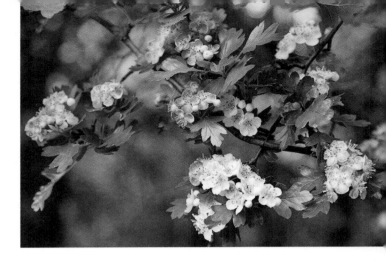

Crataegus spp.
(*C. monogyna, C. oxyacanthoides*)
Rosaceae

COMMON NAMES Hawthorn, Mayflower

PARTS USED Leaves, flowering tips (flowers and top leaves), berries.

ACTIONS Hypotensive, circulatory adaptogen, cardiac tonic, cardioprotective, vasodilator, antioxidant, astringent.

INDICATIONS High blood pressure, low blood pressure, poor circulation, palpitations, heart weakness, diarrhea, varicose veins, poor eyesight, chilblains, anxiety, stress.

DESCRIPTION A thorny shrub or small tree with bright green, lobed leaves. Its flowers are white, sometimes with a hint of pink, and appear in spring, followed by shiny, scarlet-red berries in the early autumn. It has a strong, sweetish ,and almost cloying smell when in flower.

USES Hawthorn's primary use is as a circulatory tonic; it improves blood circulation around the body and is used to treat a wide range of circulatory problems. It relaxes the coronary arteries and dilates the peripheral blood vessels to allow blood to circulate more efficiently around the body. It also supports the heart's ability to pump effectively without increasing the heart rate, making it the number one herb for high blood pressure.

Hawthorn is a circulatory adaptogen, meaning it will also help to raise blood pressure that is too low. Combine hawthorn with yarrow and linden blossom for a blood–pressure–lowering tea or tincture that can be taken daily to keep the heart and circulatory system healthy.

Hawthorn contains plant compounds called oligomeric procyanidins (OPCs) and other flavonoids. These are powerful antioxidants that relax the central nervous system, making it an excellent remedy for anxiety and stress, particularly where there is a feeling of panic and heart palpitations.

Traditionally, the berries were used medicinally. We now know that the young leaves and flowers contain even more OPCs than the berries; we combine them all in the Hawthorn Brandy recipe on page 171.

The protective effects of hawthorn span beyond the circulatory system. Because the circulatory system is responsible for delivering nutrients and oxygen all over the body, hawthorn can help many other body systems by keeping tissues well nourished and healthy. It assists even the tiniest blood vessels in the eyes and fingertips, making it a useful remedy for chilblains and bad eyesight caused by poor circulation.

The spring leaves and flowers were once a favorite snack, given the nickname of "bread and cheese"; they were nibbled straight from the tree. Although they do not taste much like bread or cheese, they have a wonderful fresh and green yet nutty flavor. The very young leaves and flowers are a lovely addition to salads. The berries can also be eaten straight from the tree, but do be careful and just nibble the flesh from the outside of the berries as inside they contain hard seeds.

In traditional Chinese medicine, the species *Crataegus pinnatifida*, or Chinese Hawthorn, is preferred and is used for IBS and other conditions of the digestive tract. The berries contain high amounts of pectin, a form of soluble fiber, which can be useful for soothing irritated tissues in the gut. An infusion of the berries or leaves is mildly astringent and is a gentle remedy for diarrhea, safe for use in children and the elderly.

HAWTHORN BRANDY

Brandy is the traditional chosen alcohol for tincturing hawthorn. This recipe uses both the autumn berries and the spring-flowering tops to extract the most circulatory-enhancing phytochemicals from the plant. Because it uses both the berries and flowering tops, this recipe is started in the autumn and finished in the spring, so you'll need to be patient, as it will be a while until it's ready to drink!

1 pound fresh hawthorn berries (collect in the autumn)
²/₃ cup light or dark brown sugar or honey (optional)
about 1 (750ml) bottle brandy
a few handfuls of fresh hawthorn
    flowering tops (collect in the spring)
Optional extras: 3 cinnamon sticks,
    10 whole cloves, finely grated zest of
    1 unwaxed orange and ½ teaspoon
    grated nutmeg

Collect the hawthorn berries in the autumn when they are ripe. Crush them slightly using a mortar and pestle. Place the berries in a sterilized, large, wide-mouthed Mason jar, pour over the sugar or honey (if using), then add any optional extras. Pour in enough brandy to cover the mixture.

Seal the jar, then label and date. Leave in a cool, dark place until the spring, shaking the jar occasionally.

In the spring, harvest the hawthorn flowering tops when the flowers are just opening, then add these to the berry mix. Cover the whole lot with more brandy, seal again, then leave to sit for an additional 1 month, shaking the jar occasionally.

After this time, strain the mixture, discard the hawthorn berries and flowering tops (and any optional extras, if used), then re-bottle the resulting elixir in sterilized bottles. Seal, label, and date.

To use, take 2 teaspoons daily. Try adding a shot of hawthorn brandy to a hot infusion for a winter drink for colds and flu.

TIP For a warming winter drink, make an infusion with boiling water, a cinnamon stick, and a few whole cloves, then pour in 2 tablespoons hawthorn brandy; add a squeeze of lemon juice and sugar or honey to taste.

SHELF LIFE Up to 2 years in a cool, dark place.

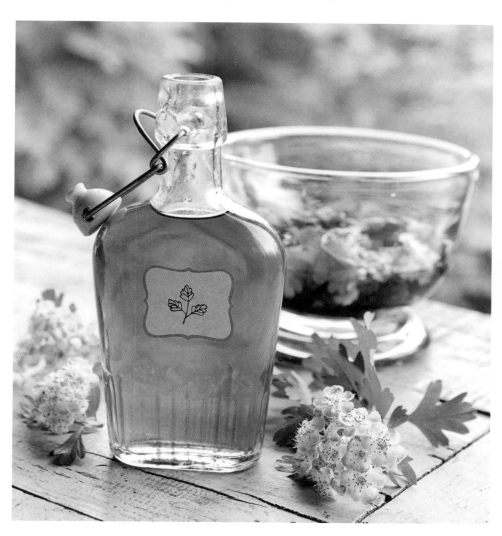

HAWTHORN FRUIT LEATHERS

To get the full benefit from hawthorn berries, make them into tasty fruit leathers. You can also use other foraged fruit; for example, bilberries, apples, blackberries, elderberries, or pears, to give them more flavor and even more of an antioxidant kick. Kids will love them too.

14 ounces fresh hawthorn berries
8 ounces (prepared weight) other mixed fresh fruits
   and berries (see intro above for examples)
1 teaspoon ground cinnamon (optional)
1–2 tablespoons honey (optional)

Preheat the oven to its lowest setting (ideally below 175°F if you can). Line 1 or 2 baking sheets with wax paper.

Place the hawthorn berries, other fruits and berries and cinnamon (if using) in a large saucepan and add 1 cup water. Bring gently to a boil, then simmer, uncovered, for about 20–30 minutes, until softened.

Remove from the heat, mash the mixture with a potato masher, then rub the pulp through a fine-mesh strainer to remove the seeds (discard the seeds in the sieve). If you are using honey, stir it into the pulp now.

Pour the pulp onto the lined baking sheet or sheets to $\frac{1}{8}$ inch thickness, spreading it evenly. Place in the oven, then leave the oven door open a crack to allow any moisture to escape. You can use a dehydrator instead if you have one.

Leave the mixture in the oven to dry; this will take anywhere between 4–8 hours, depending on the fruit used. Once dry, the pulp should be dehydrated and set but still flexible (the same kind of texture as dried fruit); once ready, it should no longer stick to your finger when touched.

Once dry, remove from the oven and transfer (still on the paper) to a wire rack to cool, then cut into strips about 1 $\frac{1}{2}$ inches wide, cutting the paper too as you go. Roll up each fruit leather strip in the wax paper for easy storage. Store in an airtight container in the fridge.

To use, eat one strip of hawthorn fruit leather a day for a healthy snack or for circulatory health.

SHELF LIFE Up to 1 month in the fridge. Alternatively, freeze the leather for up to 1 year (defrost before eating).

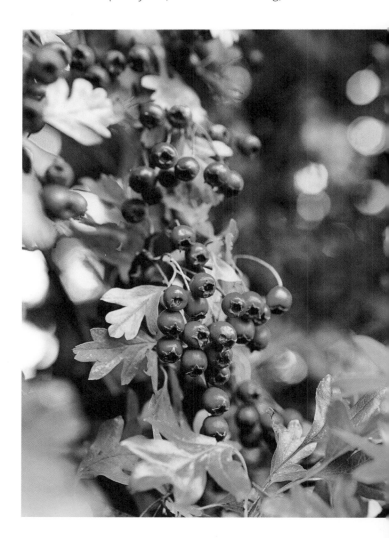

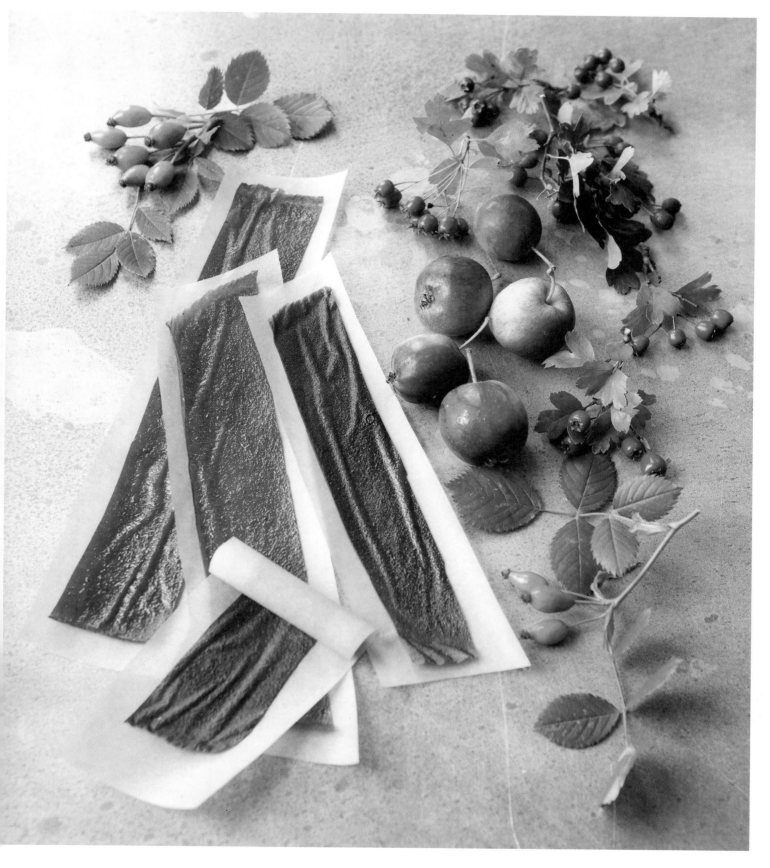

Eucalyptus globulus and other species
Myrtaceae

COMMON NAME Eucalyptus

PARTS USED Leaves, gum.

ACTIONS Antimicrobial, decongestant, antiviral.

INDICATIONS Colds, flu, coughs, respiratory congestion, topical bacterial and fungal infections.

DESCRIPTION This tall tree has a distinctive silvery bark that peels off in sheets. The mature leaves are matt green and sickle-shaped. The flower bud is covered with a cap that pops off to show a pale flower with multiple stamens and a rich honeyed scent. Harvest in spring or summer and use fresh or dried.

USES For colds, flu, coughs, and congestion, add the fresh leaves or essential oil to a bowl of hot water to create a steam inhalation. The essential oil can be added to a base cream for a decongestant effect when applied to the chest or as an antimicrobial for cuts and wounds.

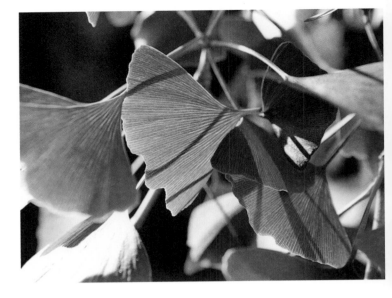

Ginkgo biloba
Ginkgoaceae

COMMON NAME Ginkgo

PARTS USED Leaves.

ACTIONS Circulatory tonic.

INDICATIONS Poor circulation, varicose veins, tinnitus, poor memory and concentration, low energy.

DESCRIPTION The ginkgo is an ancient tree dating back two hundred million years and is the sole survivor in its family. It has fan-shaped leaves with parallel veins and a slight split in the leaf, giving it the bi-lobed appearance of its Latin name. It has separate female and male plants, the females producing a strong-smelling, greenish yellow, round fruit.

USES Ginkgo is used in infusions, capsules, and tinctures to strengthen the blood vessels and encourage circulation to the extremities, warming cold hands and feet and helping to improve varicose veins. It also encourages circulation to the head and brain to improve conditions such as tinnitus, poor memory, and concentration. Harvest the leaves as they begin to turn yellow at the beginning of the autumn.

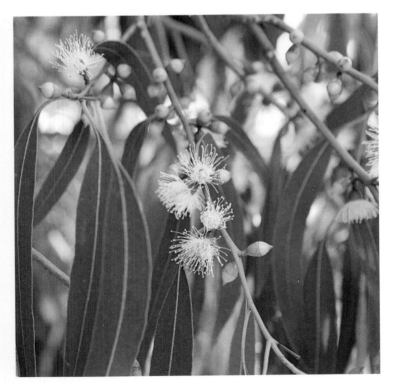

Hamamelis virginiana
Hamamelidaceae

COMMON NAME Witch Hazel

PARTS USED Bark.

ACTIONS Astringent, cooling.

INDICATIONS Inflamed skin conditions, such as bruises, varicose veins, hemorrhoids.

DESCRIPTION Witch hazel is a medium-size shrub with alternate, toothed leaves. The flowers bloom in the winter, along with the previous year's fruit, and are small with yellow, stringy petals and deep burgundy centers. The plant's strong scent is said to be citrusy by some and by others to be slightly ammonia-like.

USES Witch hazel bark is decocted to create an astringent and cooling liquid, which is used as an external wash for medicinal uses and in beauty products for oily and blemished skin. It makes an astringent, soothing compress for hot inflamed bumps, bruises and inflammation, and helps to contract varicose veins and hemorrhoids. Use the decoction in creams or lotions or simply as a refrigerated spray to cool swollen legs in hot weather.

CAUTION For external use only.

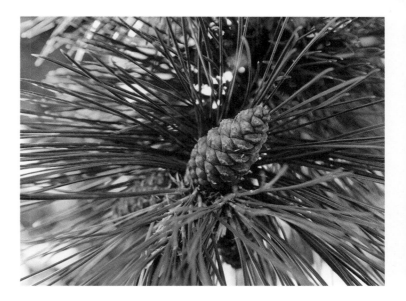

Pinus sylvestris, Pinus spp.
Pinaceae

COMMON NAMES Scots Pine, Pine Tree

PARTS USED Pine needles (leaves).

ACTIONS Antimicrobial, decongestant, circulatory.

INDICATIONS Coughs, colds, congestion, topical infections, muscle aches and pains.

DESCRIPTION Pine trees typically grow in the cooler climes of the northern hemisphere and make up many coniferous woodlands. The trees are evergreen, with long, needle-like, fresh scented leaves. The fruits are borne on pinecones.

USES The fresh, clean scent of pine needles is from its essential oils called pinenes, which are decongesting and antimicrobial. Use them in steam baths to open up the airways for coughs and respiratory congestion. The infused or essential oil of pine needles can be added to rubs and ointments to warm up achy joints and add an antimicrobial addition to first aid creams. A traditional tea made with the needles is drunk in Sweden for its vitamin C content.

CAUTION Do not mistake yew trees for pine trees, as they are toxic. Yews have short, flexible, scentless needles and the females have red berry fruits.

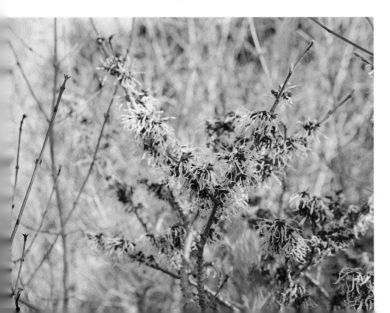

Prunus avium; P. serotina; P. padus
Rosaceae

COMMON NAMES Wild Cherry/Sweet Cherry;
Wild Black Cherry/Black Cherry; Bird Cherry

PARTS USED Inner bark from branches.

ACTIONS Antitussive.

INDICATIONS Dry, unproductive coughs.

DESCRIPTION Cherry tree bark is smooth and shiny with horizontal lines of dots called lenticels that help the tree to breathe. The leaves are oval and finely toothed. The five-petaled flowers are white or pink and are sometimes arranged in clusters or spikes, depending on the species. There are many similar species, so it is best to find a guidebook describing the differences.

USES Cherry bark helps to soothe dry painful coughs where there is no phlegm produced, especially if coughing is preventing a restful night's sleep. Harvest in autumn after the leaves drop and dry the bark for year-round use; it will keep in an airtight container in a cool, dark place for up to 1 year. Traditionally made into soothing syrups by either steeping the bark in brandy or vodka for 2 weeks, or decocting the bark for 10–15 minutes in water and simmering gently (it is said the properties are destroyed at high heat). Whichever method you choose, strain and add an equal amount of honey to the mix. The decoction method can be stored in an airtight container in the fridge for up to 1 month. The alcohol method will keep in a cool, dark place for up to 2 years.

CAUTION Do not use wild cherry bark for prolonged periods of time. The flowers and leaves contain hydrogen cyanide and should not be used.

Quercus spp.
Fagaceae

COMMON NAME Oak

PARTS USED Branch or sapling bark.

ACTIONS Astringent, styptic, antiseptic.

INDICATIONS Diarrhea, varicose veins, haemorrhoids, gingivitis.

DESCRIPTION Oaks can grow to about one thousand years old and are found all over the world, making oak an accessible medicine. The leaves are simple with rounded, wavy lobes. The fruit is an acorn, which is an oval seed that sits in a little cup-like holder (see top right).

USES The acorns have been used in the past to make a type of edible flour, but require complex processing. Medicinally, oak is a cooling and extremely astringent plant. This astringency can be used for treating and "drying-up" diarrhea, for cuts and wounds, or mixed with other herbs for gum disease. Dry the bark and powder it for infusions or tinctures to be added to creams and lotions for tightening varicose veins and hemorrhoids.

Salix alba, S. caprea
Salicaceae

COMMON NAMES White Willow, Goat Willow

PARTS USED Bark.

ACTIONS Anti-inflammatory, analgesic, febrifuge.

INDICATIONS Arthritis, rheumatism, joint pain, general pain, headaches, fever.

DESCRIPTION Tall, lithe willows like to grow near water, by the banks of rivers or over underground springs. The leaves are lanceolate and grow around the branch in a spiral arrangement. The branches have a yellowish tinge and this makes it easy to spot willows in winter. The seeds are fluffy and coat the ground in white carpets beneath the trees.

There are over four hundred species of willow and it is worth investigating your local type for traditional uses, but the white willow (*Salix alba*) and goat willow (S. *caprea*) have high amounts of salicylic acid and are most commonly used in Western herbal medicine.

USES Willow has been in use since ancient times: Hippocrates recommended its use for reducing pain and fever about 2,500 years ago. In the eighteenth century, salicylic acid was isolated from the bark, from which the anti-inflammatory painkiller aspirin was created.

Use willow bark for painful and inflamed joints, rheumatism, arthritis, and fevers for its good general pain relief and fever-reducing properties. Decoct or tincture the bitter bark for internal use, or infuse in an oil to make a balm for externally soothing joints.

CAUTION Not suitable for people sensitive to salicylates.

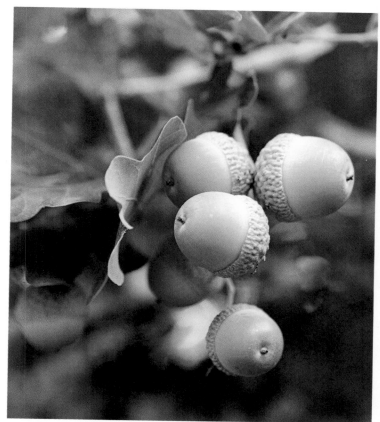

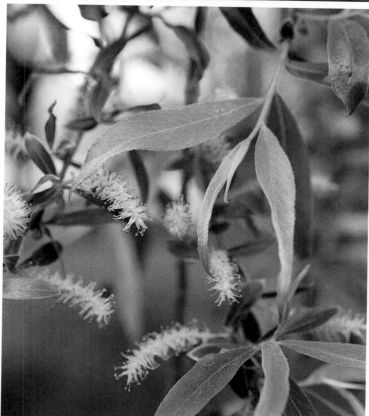

Sambucus nigra
Adoxaceae

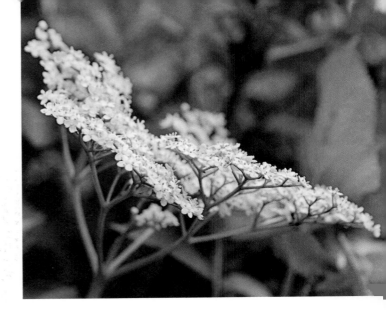

COMMON NAMES Elder, elderflower, elderberry, bore tree

PARTS USED Flowers, leaves, berries.

ACTIONS Antiviral, diaphoretic, anti-allergy, vein-strengthening.

INDICATIONS
LEAVES (topically) Aches, bruises, sprains.
FLOWERS Hay fever, sinusitis, colds, flu.
BERRIES Viral and bacterial infections, colds, flu, sore throats, coughs.

DESCRIPTION Smaller than a tree but larger than a shrub, elder can grow up to 24 feet in height. Its opposite leaves are bright green and pinnate with 5–9 ovate, toothed leaflets. The bark is light gray with the young branches having small dark holes speckled over them. The flowers are cream, sometimes with a hint of pink, and are displayed in large flat clusters. They have a sharp but sweet smell that some love and others dislike. The round berries are borne on the stems after the flowers die back, starting out green and becoming shiny, purple-black as they ripen toward the end of summer.

USES An old saying goes "summer has not arrived until elderflower is in full bloom and ends when the berries are ripe". The elder can be found in many a park or field, famed for its aromatic flowers, which make delicious cordials and champagnes. Like many medicinal plants, its prevalence and plentiful folklore indicates its usefulness; elder is a medicine cabinet in its own right. In fact, the elder is held in such reverence that legend says you must ask permission from the resident Elder Mother before picking!

The leaves, stems, and raw or unripe berries of elder contain a mildly toxic cyanoglycoside, which if taken internally, can induce vomiting. The leaves and stems were once used as an emetic to purge the body of "vile ills." Cooking, tincturing or drying the berries destroys the toxic compounds, rendering them edible, medicinal, and tasty.

The leaves are some of the first to appear after winter and are infused in oils and ointments to treat bruising, sore muscles, and chilblains. They contain sambunigrin, which when applied topically, relieves pain.

In the spring, elder supplies us with an abundance of creamy white flowers, high in flavonoids, rutin, and isoquercitrin. These compounds are anti-inflammatory and anti-allergic and specifically act to soothe inflamed tissues in the upper respiratory tract and sinuses — just in time for hay fever season! A great remedy for colds and flu, elderflower is slightly antiviral and it dries up excess mucus and brings down a fever by encouraging sweating. A traditional way to break a fever in colds or flu was to have hot elderflower infusion, go to bed, and sweat profusely.

Elderflowers are best harvested on a sunny day when their fragrance, flavor and chemical constituents are at their peak.

In the autumn, we are rewarded with a bountiful harvest of purple-black berries. These are high in vitamins A and C, flavonoids, and antioxidants. Studies have shown the berries to be an effective antiviral, preventing cold and flu viruses from replicating. They also act as an immune booster, keeping the immune system healthy and ready to fight off infection. The berries freeze well and make a tasty and immune-boosting addition to pies, oatmeal and crumbles.

ELDERBERRY SYRUP

Delicious spiced elderberry syrup can be added to hot infusions to soothe sore throats and coughs during winter illness. It can also be used at the first signs of infection to strengthen the immune system.

1 pound fresh elderberries
2 cinnamon sticks
3 star anise
1 inch piece of fresh ginger, sliced
10 cardamom pods
5 whole cloves
1 teaspoon dried unwaxed orange peel
unrefined sugar (superfine or granulated)

Place the elderberries, spices and orange peel in a saucepan, then pour over 500ml water. Bring to a boil over medium heat, then simmer, uncovered, for 20–30 minutes, stirring occasionally, until the liquid has reduced slightly.

Remove from the heat and leave to cool, then strain the liquid through a piece of cheesecloth set over a bowl, to remove the seeds. Thoroughly squeeze the juice from the berries.

Measure the liquid and return to the cleaned pan, then add the same amount of sugar (so you have equal parts juice to sugar, i.e. for every 1 cup of liquid, add 1 cup of sugar.). Bring slowly to a boil, stirring until the sugar has dissolved, then simmer gently for 10–15 minutes until reduced and thickened.

Pour the hot syrup into sterilized bottles, seal, label and date.

To use, take 2–4 teaspoons in a little water or add to a hot infusion for a warming drink.

SHELF LIFE Keep (unopened) in a cool, dark place for up to 6 months. Once opened, keep in the fridge and use within 2 weeks.

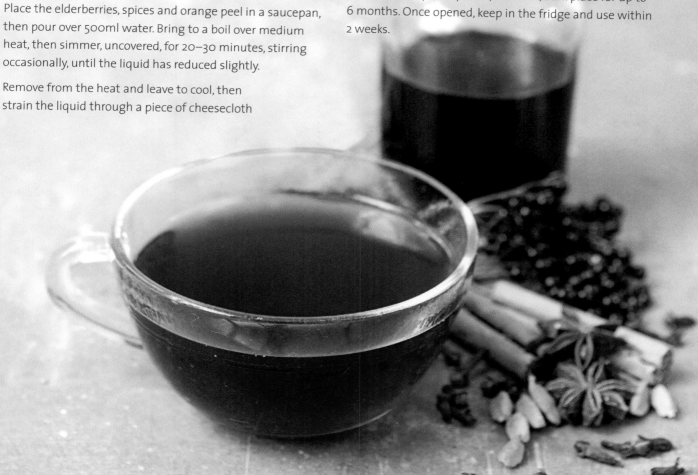

ELDERFLOWER CORDIAL

This delicious cordial epitomizes summer. It is made slightly differently from regular syrups, in that the flowers are infused at the end of the process to preserve their delicate flavor. Use in cold drinks or add to hot water to make a diaphoretic brew for winter ills.

5 cups unrefined sugar (caster or granulated)
20 heads of fresh elderflowers
   (enough to fill a large colander)
2 tablespoons citric acid
finely grated zest and juice of 2 lemons

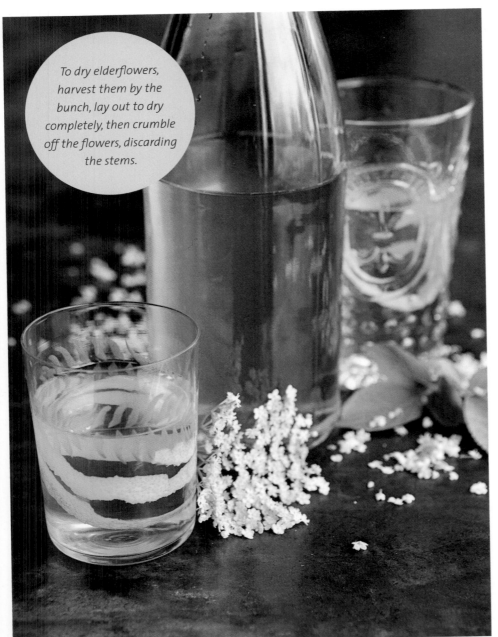

To dry elderflowers, harvest them by the bunch, lay out to dry completely, then crumble off the flowers, discarding the stems.

Pour 1 ½ quarts water into a saucepan and bring to a boil, then add the sugar and stir until dissolved. Bring to a boil again, then reduce the heat and simmer for 5–10 minutes, until thickened to a syrup. Remove from the heat.

Remove the flowers from their stems with a fork (making sure you've rescued any bugs that are on the flowers). Add the flowers, citric acid, and lemon zest and juice to the sugar syrup and stir to combine.

Transfer the mix to a large jar or glass bowl and cover with a clean cloth. Leave for 1 day, stirring once or twice.

Strain through cheesecloth into a bowl, then pour into sterilized bottles, seal, label, and date.

To use, mix 1 part cordial to 3–4 parts still or sparkling water. In the winter, try it with hot water.

SHELF LIFE Keep (unopened) in a cool, dark place for up to 6 months. Once opened, keep in the fridge and use within 2 weeks. Alternatively, freeze the cordial in ice cube trays or plastic bottles for up to 1 year (defrost before serving).

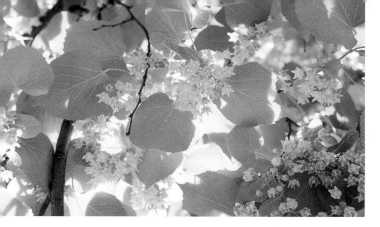

Tilia spp. *(T. cordata, T. platyphyllos, T. x europaea)*
Malvaceae

COMMON NAMES Linden or Lime (small-leaved, large-leaved, common)

PARTS USED Flowers, bracts, and youngest leaves growing nearest to the flowers.

ACTIONS Hypotensive, anti-anxiety, hypocholesterolemic.

INDICATIONS Insomnia, anxiety, stress, high cholesterol, high blood pressure, palpitations, migraines.

DESCRIPTION The linden tree has pretty heart-shaped leaves that are pale green in the spring but darken over summer. *Tilia x europaea* is commonly planted along streets and can be recognized by numerous green shoots that sprout from the base of the trunk. The flowers are unusual, with a large, green, strap-like bract that acts as a sail for the ripened seeds. They protrude from this bract on a long stalk and pop open a crown of stamens that give out a rich, pervading, honeyed scent. Pick the flowers and bracts within a week of blooming when the stamens are still fresh and sticky.

USES Many countries in Europe sell traditional herbal tea made from the tasty flowers of linden for relaxation and insomnia. It is particularly effective for children, and an infusion can be used as a bath to help send them off to sleep. Linden is used as an effective cardiotonic — it lowers high blood pressure and reduces cholesterol. Infusions also soothe and calm the nerves in cases of anxiety associated with heart palpitations and some types of migraines.

Viburnum opulus
Adoxaceae

COMMON NAMES Crampbark, Guelder Rose

PARTS USED Bark.

ACTIONS Antispasmodic, astringent.

INDICATIONS Period pain, muscle spasms, digestive spasms, tension headaches.

DESCRIPTION Crampbark is a small shrub/tree with palmate leaves, attractive flowers, and berries. The flowers are clustered in a flat head with inconspicuous inner flowers and an outer circle of larger white-petaled ones, similar to hydrangea. The autumn berries form as bright orangey red clusters.

USES Crampbark does what its name says: it is used as a muscle relaxant for cramps. This is helpful for any muscle tension and spasm, including menstrual pain and leg cramps. This relaxant property can also work in a sedative manner for nervous tension. The bark is harvested after the plant drops its leaves and before the following year's buds develop. This makes it easy to strip off the branch. Dry the bark for tincturing or powdering for capsules.

CAUTION Not suitable for people sensitive to salicylates.

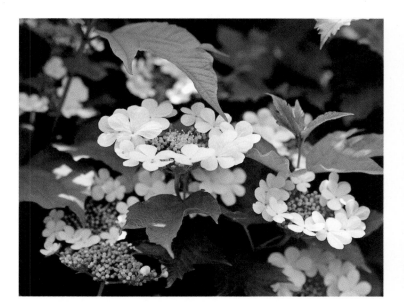

COMMON NAME AND LATIN NAME CHECKLIST

Aloe — *Aloe vera*

Angelica — *Angelica archangelica*

Balm, lemon — *Melissa officinalis*

Basil — *Ocimum basilicum*

Berberis — *Berberis vulgaris, B. aquifolium*

Birch, silver — *Betula pendula*

Blackberry — *Rubus fruticosus*

Bramble — *Rubus fruticosus*

Broadleaf plantain — *Plantago major*

Burdock — *Arctium lappa*

Calendula — *Calendula officinalis*

Californian poppy — *Eschscholzia californica*

Chamomile — *Matricaria chamomilla, Chamaemelum nobile*

Chickweed — *Stellaria media*

Chicory — *Cichorium intybus*

Chile/chile pepper — *Capsicum spp.*

Cinnamon — *Cinnamomum spp.*

Cleavers — *Galium aparine*

Clover, red — *Trifolium pratense*

Comfrey — *Symphytum officinale*

Cone flower — *Echinacea angustifolia, E. purpurea*

Corn silk — *Zea mays*

Crampbark or guelder rose — *Viburnum opulus*

Crow Garlic — *Allium vineale*

Curly or curled dock — *Rumex crispus*

Daisy — *Bellis perennis*

Dandelion — *Taraxacum officinale*

Dill — *Anethum graveolens*

Dock — *Rumex crispus*

Echinacea — *Echinacea angustifolia, E. purpurea*

Elder — *Sambucus nigra*

Elecampane — *Inula helenium*

Eucalyptus — *Eucalyptus globulus, E. smithii, E. polybractea, E. radiata*

Fennel — *Foeniculum vulgare*

Feverfew — *Tanacetum parthenium*

Garlic — *Allium sativum*

Garlic mustard — *Allaria petiolata*

German chamomile — *Matricaria chamomilla*

Ginger — *Zingiber officinale*

Ginkgo — *Ginkgo biloba*

Goosegrass — *Galium aparine*

Ground ivy — *Glechoma hederacea*

Herb robert — *Geranium robertianum*

Hoary plantain — *Plantago media*

Honeysuckle — *Lonicera periclymenum, L. caprifolium*

Horse chestnut — *Aesculus hippocastanum*

Horsetail — *Equisetum arvense*

Juniper — *Juniperus communis*

Lady's mantle — *Alchemilla vulgaris, A. mollis*

Lavender — *Lavandula angustifolia*

Lemon balm — *Melissa officinalis*

Linden/Lime — *Tilia cordata, T. platyphyllos, T. x europaea*

Licorice — *Glycyrrhiza glabra*

Mahonia — *Berberis aquifolium*

Mallow, common — *Malva sylvestris*

Marshmallow — *Althaea officinalis*

Meadowsweet — *Filipendula ulmaria*

Melissa — *Melissa officinalis*

Milk thistle — *Silybum marianum*

Mint — *Mentha spp.*

Motherwort — *Leonurus cardiaca*

Mullein — *Verbascum thapsus*

Mustard — *Brassica alba, B. nigra*

Nettle — *Urtica dioica*

Oak — *Quercus spp.*

Oats, oat straw — *Avena sativa*

Oregano — *Origanum vulgare* (oregano/wild marjoram), *O. majorana* (sweet marjoram)

Oregon mountain grape — *Berberis aquifolium*

Parsley — *Petroselinum crispum, P. sativum*

Pine — *Pinus sylvestris* (Scots pine), *P. spp.* (pine tree)

Plantain — *Plantago lanceolata, P. major, P. media*

Poppy — *Papaver rhoeas, Eschscholzia californica*

Pot marigold — *Calendula officinalis*

Purple cone flower — *Echinacea angustifolia, E. purpurea*

Ramsons — *Allium Ursinum*

Raspberry — *Rubus idaeus*

Red clover — *Trifolium pratense*

Ribwort plantain — *Plantago lanceolata*

Roman chamomile — *Chamaemelum nobile*

Rose / Rosehip — *Rosa spp.*

Rosemary — *Rosmarinus officinalis*

Sage — *Salvia officinalis*

Selfheal — *Prunella vulgaris*

Shepherd's purse — *Capsella bursa-pastoris*

Skullcap — *Scutellaria lateriflora*

Sticky willy — *Galium aparine*

Stinging nettle — *Urtica dioica*

St John's wort — *Hypericum perforatum*

Sweet Corn — *Zea mays*

Three-cornered leek — *Allium triquetrum*

Thyme — *Thymus vulgaris*

Turmeric — *Curcuma longa*

Vervain — *Verbena officinalis*

Violet — *Viola odorata*

Wild cherry — *Prunus avium* (wild cherry/sweet cherry), *P. serotina* (wild black cherry), *P. padus* (bird cherry)

Wild garlic — *Allium ursinum*

Wild leek — *Allium triquetrum*

Wild lettuce — *Lactuca virosa*

Willow — *Salix alba, S. caprea*

Witch hazel — *Hamamelis virginiana*

Wood betony — *Stachys officinalis*

Yarrow — *Achillea millefolium*

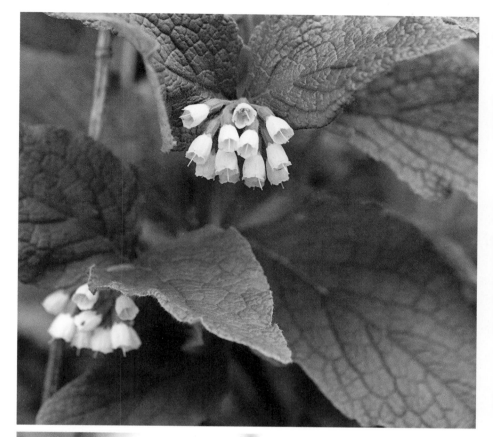

Comfrey *Symphytum officinale* (top) and Three-cornered leek *Allium triquetrum* (bottom)

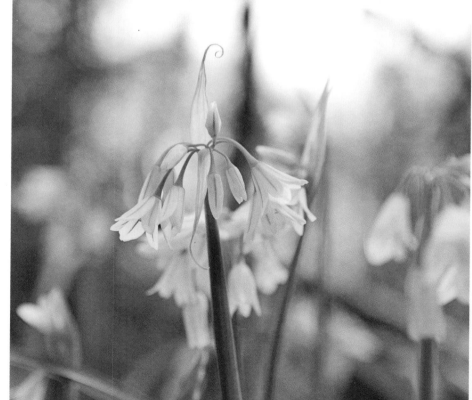

GLOSSARY

ADAPTOGEN — An herb that helps to increase resilience to stress
and disease (see page 54 for a more in-depth discussion)

AERIAL PARTS — The upper parts of a flowering plant before it has gone to seed. These include the leaves, flowers, and non-woody stems.

ALTERATIVES — Herbs used as blood cleansers; see page 54 for their action on specific body systems.

AMENORRHOEA — Abnormal absence of menstruation.

ANALGESIC — Reduces or relieves pain.

ANTI-ALLERGIC — Helps to alleviate some symptoms of allergy, such as hay fever.

ANTIARTHRITIC — Lessens symptoms of arthritis.

ANTIBACTERIAL — Destroys or inhibits the growth of bacteria.

ANTICOAGULANT — Inhibits blood coagulation (clotting). Some prescription drugs are anticoagulent, so if you are receiving these drugs, please seek advice before taking herbs in conjunction with them.

ANTIEMETIC — Lessens or stops nausea and vomiting.

ANTIFUNGAL — Inhibits or prevents fungal infection.

ANTIHISTAMINE — Histamine is a chemical produced by the body and is involved in immune and inflammatory response. It is usually overactive in allergic conditions such as hay fever. Antihistamines help to regulate this response.

ANTIHYDROTIC — Reduces or prevents excess perspiration.

ANTI-INFECTIVE/ANTIMICROBIAL — Destroys or prevents the growth of microorganisms such as viruses, bacteria, fungi, and parasites.

ANTI-INFLAMMATORY — Reduces inflammation.

ANTI-ITCH — Stops or soothes itching.

ANTIOXIDANT — Prevents oxidative stress from free radicals, thus preventing damage to cells and tissues.

ANTIPARASITIC — Treats parasites.

ANTIPYRETIC — Reduces fever.

ANTIRHEUMATIC — Reduces the symptoms of rheumatism.

ANTISEPTIC — Antimicrobial (see also Anti-infective entry above).

ANTISPASMODIC — Reduces spasms, usually in the muscles, helping to relax tension and cramping.

ANTITUSSIVE — Suppresses the cough reflex.

ANTIVIRAL — Prevents or inhibits viral infections.

ANXIOLYTIC/ANTI-ANXIETY — Reduces anxiety.

APERITIF — A pre- or post-meal drink to stimulate appetite and improve digestion.

AROMATIC — Strong-smelling herbs that contain volatile oils. These can relieve muscular spasm and spasm of the gut. They can reduce digestive discomfort and wind. Usually antimicrobial.

ASTRINGENT — Tightens tissues by causing proteins in tissues to contract. They can relieve inflammation and reduce secretions, discharges and bleeding.

AUTOIMMUNE — A disorder where the body's immune system attacks or damages the body's own healthy cells and tissues.

AYURVEDA/AYURVEDIC — An Indian traditional healing system that also uses herbs.

BAIN-MARIE — A hot water bath or double boiler, used to gently infuse or cook foods or herbs (see the "How to Infuse Your Oil" section on page 22 in the Make section for further instructions on this).

BIOAVAILABILITY —A chemical or substance that is able to be absorbed into the body and have an effect.

BITTER — Herbs that taste bitter; they stimulate digestive juices and improve overall digestion.

CARDIAC AND CIRCULATORY TONIC — Strengthens the heart and blood vessels.

CARDIOPROTECTIVE — Protects the heart and circulatory system.

CARMINATIVE — Herbs that contain aromatic compounds; these aid digestion and reduce digestive discomfort from spasm and wind.

CONSTITUENT — A component of a whole; in this case a chemical within a plant.

COUNTER-IRRITANT — Something that produces a surface irritation to the skin, increasing blood circulation to the area and helping to counteract pain and inflammation.

DECONGESTANT — Relieves congestion, usually catarrh, of the respiratory system.

DEMULCENT — Mucilage-rich herb that soothes inflammation.

DIAPHORETIC — Promotes sweating to reduce high fever and eliminate wastes through the pores.

DIGESTIVE — Improves or encourages normal digestion.

DIURETIC — Encourages the production of urine.

EMMENAGOGUE — Stimulates menstruation; used where bleeding is scanty or menstruation is delayed.

EMOLLIENT — Cream that increases skin hydration, both by directly moisturizing and acting as a barrier to prevent moisture loss.

EXPECTORANT — Supports the removal of excess mucus and catarrh of the respiratory system.

FEBRIFUGE — Reduces fever.

GALACTAGOGUE — An herb or food that encourages milk production in mothers.

GENUS / GENERA — a taxonomic rank used to classify groups of plants.

HEPATOPROTECTIVE — Protects the liver.

HYPERTENSIVE — Increases blood pressure (hypertensive herbs are sometimes useful in conditions of low blood pressure).

HYPOCHOLESTEROLEMIC — Blood lipid lowering; used for high cholesterol.

HYPOTENSIVE — Lowers blood pressure.

IMMUNE MODULATOR — Modulates or regulates immune function.

IMMUNE STIMULANT — Stimulates aspects of the immune system.

LAXATIVE — Stimulates bowel movement.

LYMPHATIC — Supports lymphatic function. Used to support the body where there is infection or stagnation. Aids in detoxification.

MUCILAGE/MUCILAGINOUS — Complex carbohydrate molecules found in plants that have a gelatinous, gloopy consistency.

MUCOLYTIC — Thins and breaks down mucus.

NERVINE — Nerve tonic; relaxes and soothes physical and emotional stress.

NUTRITIVE — Provides nourishment.

PELVIC DECONGESTANT — Encourages circulation of the pelvic region.

PHYTOCHEMICAL — Naturally occurring plant chemicals.

POLYCYSTIC OVARIAN SYNDROME (PCOS) — A hormonal condition characterised by many cysts on the ovaries.

RELAXANT — Muscle or tissue relaxing.

RE-MINERALISER — An herb high in vitamins and minerals that can be used to boost nutrition.

RUBEFACIENT — Increases local circulation to the skin.

SEDATIVE — Relaxes the nervous system and encourages sleep.

STIMULANT — An herb that increases or encourages a function, for example, a 'digestive stimulant' encourages normal digestion in cases where it is underactive or slow.

STYPTIC — An astringent herb that reduces bleeding.

SYMPTOMATIC — In herbal terms, this may mean working to treat the symptoms of a disease or illness in the short-term, but may not treat the underlying problem or cause.

TONIC — Strengthens and supports a system or organ.

VASODILATOR — Relaxes and dilates the veins and arteries.

VULNERARY — Promotes wound healing.

WARMING — Has a heating effect on an organ, system or throughout the body, usually through increasing circulation.

HERBAL FIRST AID KIT

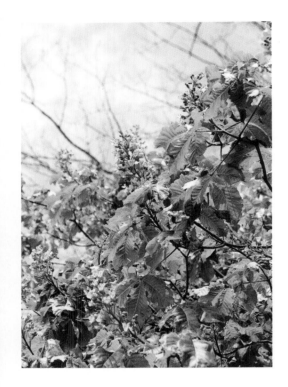

A well-stocked herbal first aid kit is essential to have on hand for when illness strikes. Here are ten remedies to keep in the first aid box or travel kit:

ST. JOHN'S WORT- OR CALENDULA-INFUSED OIL — rashes, cuts, bites, burns (see page 22 for infused oils).

COMFREY AND ELDER BALM— bruising, joint and muscle pain and injury (see page 61).

ANTI-ALLERGY TEA — hay fever, eczema, general allergies, sinus infections (see page 80).

MEADOWSWEET AND MILK THISTLE SOOTHING LOZENGES — vomiting, diarrhea, indigestion, convalescence, heartburn, sore throat, hangovers (see page 141).

SOOTHING SKIN CREAM — eczema, psoriasis, wounds (see page 72).

ELDERBERRY SYRUP — coughs, colds, sore throats, general infections (see page 179).

LAVENDER ESSENTIAL OIL— steam inhalations, sinus congestion, respiratory infection, insomnia, burns, wounds, headaches.

HAWTHORN BRANDY— insomnia, anxiety, high blood pressure, colds, flu (see page 171).

BITTER DIGESTIVE DROPS — indigestion, constipation, nausea, hangovers (see page 45).

IMMUNE TONIC TINCTURE — general infections of all kinds (see page 57).

FINDING AN HERBALIST

RESOURCES

THE AMERICAN ASSOCIATION OF NATUROPATHIC PHYSICIANS (AANP)

818 18th St. NW
Suite 250
Washington, DC 20006

Telephone: 202-237-8150

THE AMERICAN HERBALISTS GUILD (AHG)

PO. Box 3076
Asheville, NC 28802-3076

Telephone: 617-520-4372
office@americanherbalistsguild.com

There are many suppliers of herbal products and ingredients all over the US, but please check the members directory of the American Herbal Products Association (AHPA) (www.ahpa.org) who promote industry standards regarding safety and sustainability.

MOUNTAIN ROSE HERBS
Suppliers of organic, sustainable herbs and remedy ingredients.

PO Box 50220
Eugene, OR 97405
www.mountainroseherbs.com
support@mountainroseherbs.
comtarwest-botanicals.com
Telephone: (800) 879-3337 or
(541) 741-7307

STARWEST BOTANICALS
Herbs, oils & remedy ingredients.

161 Main Ave.
Sacramento, CA, 95838
www.starwest-botanicals.com
Telephone: 1-800-800-4372 or
(916) 638-8100

OREGON'S WILD HARVEST
Herb supplier.

1601 NE Hemlock Ave.
Redmond, OR 97756
www.oregonswildharvest.com
Telephone: (541) 548-9400
Toll Free: (800) 316-6869

FRONTIER CO-OP
Herb supplier.

PO Box 299
3021 78th St.
Norway, IA 52318
www.frontiercoop.com
customercare@frontiercoop.com
Telephone: 1-844-550-6200

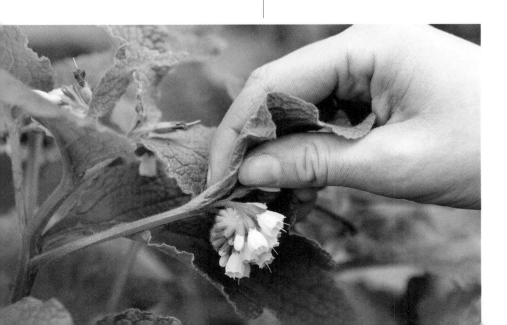

INDEX

THANK YOUS

First, to the team at Kyle books including Kyle Cathie and Judith Hannam for asking us to write this book. A special thanks to Sophie Allen for being a supportive and fantastic editor. The shoot days were so much fun and produced wonderful photography, so we are indebted to the skills of Sarah Cuttle. Thank you to Wei Tang for prop styling and Megan Smith for the design. Thank you to our agent Josie Pearse of Pearse & Black for all your support and advice.

Thanks to Diane and Peter Anderson for opening their beautiful home and herb gardens to us and supplying us with homemade scones. And to Jason Irving for his support in overlooking the finished draft. Thank you Liz Lafferty for all your help.

We couldn't have done it without you all.

VICKY CHOWN practices as a medical herbalist in London. She worked at Neal's Yard Remedies for 6 years providing natural health and beauty advice.

KIM WALKER works in environmental education and historical plant research. She is a researcher at the Royal Botanic Gardens, Kew.

Vicky and Kim met 5 years ago while studying Herbal Medicine at Westminster University. They set up Handmade Apothecary to share their passion about the natural power of plants to others.

Design Ketchup
Photographer Sarah Cuttle
Prop Stylist Wei Tang
Project Editor Sophie Allen
Editorial Assistant Hannah Coughlin
Production Nic Jones, Gemma John and Lisa Pinnell
Color reproduction by f1, London.

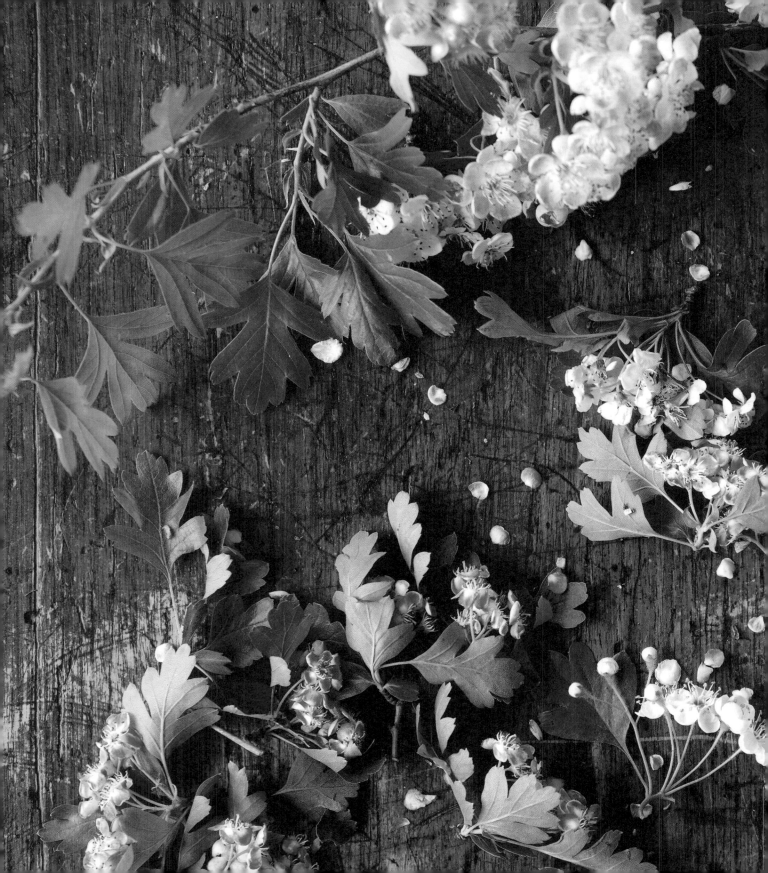